ELEVATE

50 DAYS TO TRANSFORMATION

WORKBOOK AND JOURNAL

A Guided Journey to Raise Your Frequency, Rewire
Your Mind, and Become the Next Best Version of You

PROGRAM CREATED BY DOCTOR EAST

"Thoughts become things. If you see it in your mind, you will hold it in your hand."

Bob Proctor

Elevate: 50-Days to Transformation Workbook and Journal
A Guided Journey to Raise Your Frequency, Rewire Your Mind,
and Become the Next Best Version of You

979-8-9916689 4 1

For more information on Doctor East Phillips, DAOM, visit https://www.DoctorEast.com

For more information on the publisher, visit https://www.IlluminisPublishing.com

ABOUT DOCTOR EAST

Doctor East is an alternative and integrative healthcare practitioner, educator, fitness professional, and author with more than three decades of experience helping people transform their lives—physically, mentally, emotionally, and spiritually.

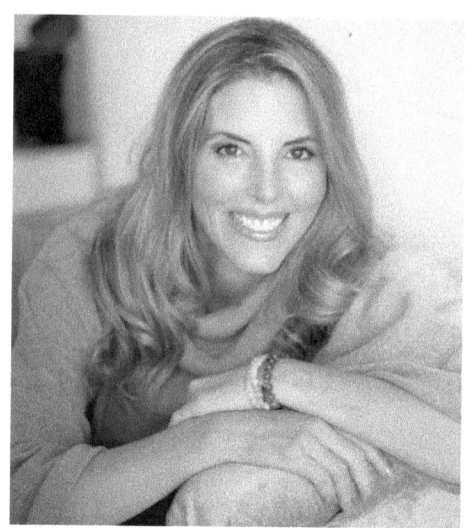

The **Elevate: 50 Days to Transformation** program is the result of decades spent in private practice, teaching at the master's and doctoral level, leading fitness classes, and working closely with thousands of individuals seeking real, lasting change. Through this work, she observed a powerful truth: true transformation happens when mindset, body, identity, habits, and purpose are addressed together—consistently and compassionately.

Doctor East has taught and mentored students at advanced levels of healthcare education, guided clients through deep personal growth in one-on-one and group settings, and remained actively engaged as a health and fitness instructor for over 30 years. This unique blend of clinical insight, academic rigor, embodied movement, and lived experience informs every page of this workbook.

She is also the author of the following books: Living Life in Your PJs: How to Stay Aligned with Your Purpose, Passion, and Joy, Decades: Reflections of a Life Well Lived Workbook and Journal, More Than a Treatment: How to Create Exceptional Experiences that Increase Patient Satisfaction and Improve Treatment Outcomes, 21 Days to Love (co-author), Natural Tools for Wellbeing, and the children's book The Rainbow Fairies: A Field Guide.

Through her programs, books, and live experiences, Doctor East is devoted to helping people remember who they really are, reconnect with their innate strength and wisdom, and maximize their experience of life.

"What you seek is seeking you."
RUMI

ABOUT THE ELEVATE PROGRAM

Elevate: 50 Days to Transformation is more than a workbook and journal. It is part of a larger, guided experience known as the Elevate Program, created by Doctor East.

The Elevate Program was developed over the course of nearly three decades of working with individuals in private practice and teaching health, wellness, and fitness. Through years of hands-on experience supporting people physically, mentally, emotionally, and spiritually, Doctor East observed a consistent truth:

Lasting transformation happens when structure, mindset, movement, language, and daily habits work together.

Why 50 Days?

The 50-day structure of Elevate is intentional and tested.

Over years of working with individuals and groups, Doctor East observed that longer programs, while well-intentioned, often lead to burnout — with most people disengaging or quitting around the 50-day mark. On the other hand, shorter programs, while motivating at first, often don't provide enough time for real integration, identity shifts, and lasting change.

Fifty days emerged as the sweet spot:

- Long enough to create meaningful habit change and internal alignment
- Structured enough to build consistency and self-trust
- Short enough to remain sustainable, engaging, and achievable

This balance allows participants to experience real momentum — not just motivation — and to carry what they've learned well beyond the program itself.

How This Workbook Fits In

This workbook & journal is designed to be a tangible companion to the Elevate experience — a place to reflect, track, write, and integrate what you are practicing day by day. While it can be used on its own, it was intentionally created to align with the Elevate Program, where participants receive guided instruction, accountability, and more coaching.

If you feel called to go deeper, expand your experience, or be guided through the 50-day journey with added structure and support, you can learn more about the full Elevate offerings — including digital programs and live events — by visiting:

www.DoctorEast.com

Thank you for allowing this work to support your journey.
May these pages serve as a place of clarity, commitment, and meaningful transformation.

TABLE OF CONTENTS

WELCOME

You have desires on your heart. Dreams. Goals. Wishes and wants. You would not be given these things without also being given the ability to manifest them into your reality.

This 50-day challenge was created to initiate the internal and external transformations required to bring you closer to obtaining your desires.

By raising your frequency you will become a magnet for more of the good things in life. More happiness, more money, more love, more health, more wealth, joy, inner peace, grounding and even more miracles.

I do not believe you found this workbook by accident. Perhaps your higher self called it into your life. Maybe God/the Universe/Source/Creator/Infinite Intelligence sent it to you to use as a tool to finally receive all of things for which you have been praying and asking. Either way, if you follow this program for fifty days straight you WILL raise your frequency. You WILL see incredible transformation in your life. You WILL begin to live a life of your dreams AND if you continue to practice and implement what is outlined in these fifty days you just may find yourself living a life beyond your wildest imagination. A life abundant in HAPPINESS, LOVE, WEALTH, HEALTH, JOY, PASSION, PURPOSE and GROWTH, EXPANSION and AWARENESS.

The path of a thousand miles begins with one step. So let's begin our journey together. You are not alone. You are never alone. Within this program you will be asked to spend time alone so that you may connect with God/infinite intelligence. The idea here is to draw on the higher power that is all around us, permeates us and co-creates life with us. A name does not matter as it would never give it justice. Refer to this higher power however you like and in a way that makes you feel supported, loved and empowered.

I have been a healthcare provider for nearly three decades now and one thing I have learned in all this time is that when we raise our frequency, everything in our lives improves. That is the first "why" behind me creating this program, workbook and journal. The second "why" is this: Imagine a world where EVERYONE worked on raising THEIR frequency. Rather than spending energy, attention and capacity on negative things like criticism, comparison and judgement, everyone spent their energy, attention and capacity on raising their frequency. Imagine a world like that. How high can we go? Let's find out. It all starts with you. It starts with me. It starts with each of us doing the work ourselves. I'm committed to living a high-frequency life and continuing to raise the collective frequency. Are you? If so, enter your commitment on the next page and join the movement.

With love & gratitude,
Doctor East

COMMITMENT TO THE NEXT
BEST VERSION OF YOURSELF

I commit to becoming the highest version of myself—physically, mentally, emotionally, and spiritually.

I devote myself to this journey of growth and self-mastery, choosing each day to show up with intention, awareness, and care. I commit to practices that support my health, strengthen my mindset, expand my emotional capacity, and deepen my spiritual connection. Through this process, I choose to live with greater clarity, compassion, and purpose—and to bring my best self into the world.

I begin this program on the date next to my signature below and commit to completing it in full. I understand that growth is not about perfection, but about consistency, honesty, and returning to what matters. If I encounter challenges or miss a day, I recommit and continue forward with self-respect and determination.

The healthy nutrition plan I intend on following is (include any special nutrition challenges you may incorporate into the 50 days like no fried foods, processed sugar, ice-cream, etc.):

_____

I am committed to this process.
I am committed to myself.
I look forward to the growth, strength, and transformation that will unfold as I walk this path.

Date: _____

Name Printed: _____

Signature:

Accountability Partner(s)
Having an accountability partner can be super helpful in this process. Identify one or more accountability partner(s) below and be grateful for them as they are part of your transformation.

Accountability partner(s):

ELEVATE: 50-DAY PROGRAM AT-A-GLANCE CHECKLIST

Day	Date	30 Min Strength Training	30 Min Movement Outside	Read 10 pages or listen to 30 min. of personal development/ growth	Follow a High Freq Nutrition	Appreciation sent out to someone	10+ min alone connection time	Gratitude & Journal Entries Complete
1								
2								
3								
4								
5								
6								
7								
8								
9								
10								
11								
12								
13								
14								
15								
16								
17								
18								
19								
20								
21								
22								
23								
24								
25								

ELEVATE: 50-DAY PROGRAM AT-A-GLANCE CHECKLIST

Day	Date	30 Min Strength Training	30 Min Movement Outside	Read 10 pages or listen to 30 min. of personal development/ growth	Follow a High Freq Nutrition	Appreciation sent out to someone	10+ min alone connection time	Gratitude & Journal Entries Complete
26								
27								
28								
29								
30								
31								
32								
33								
34								
35								
36								
37								
38								
39								
40								
41								
42								
43								
44								
45								
46								
47								
48								
49								
50								

RULES

I have a bracelet with letter beads that reads: Y.N.T.B.O.M. That stands for "You're Not The Boss of Me," so you can imagine I'm not a big fan of rigid rules. But here's the truth: a little structure goes a long way when it comes to transformation. Boundaries and consistency don't box you in—they create a sacred container for growth, expansion, and accomplishment.

So here's the deal. This program is designed as a 50-day journey, and while it's not about perfection, you'll get the most out of it if you show up every single day and complete each exercise, activity, and reflection without skipping steps or days. Each one builds upon the last, like rungs on a ladder that leads to the next best version of you. There are no "cheat days," but life happens—so if you miss a day, simply acknowledge it and recommit the next day. The magic is in the momentum. Remember, it's called a challenge for a reason: it's meant to stretch you, awaken you, and support your evolution. So show up fully. Trust the process. And let the 50 days change you in ways you can't yet imagine.

Every day for fifty days straight, you get to do these 7 Frequency Raising Activities:

1. Follow a healthy nutrition plan of your choice, abstaining from alcohol
2. Journaling
3. Express appreciation to someone
4. 10 minutes of meditation, prayer, connection to God/Infinite Intelligence/Higher Power
5. Two 30-miniute workouts (one outside and one strength training)
6. Read 10 pages or listen to 30 minutes of personal development/growth content
7. Complete the daily reflection assignment in your journal

How to use this workbook and journal
The at-a-glance checklist provided in this workbook and journal will help you ensure that you do each of the seven activities every day. You may do the activities in any order you see fit for planning out your day. All activities must be done in that day. You cannot work out for 90 minutes one day and tell yourself that 30 of those minutes are for tomorrow. You cannot read 20 pages of personal development content and tell yourself that 10 pages are for tomorrow. You cannot give appreciation to three people on one day and count it for the next three days. Every day the 7 Frequency Raising Activities are a minimum. Small tiny habits performed consistently are what initiate lasting transformation. Now, you can choose to do more of each activity on any given day. However, extra activity does not roll over like minutes on a cell phone plan.

High-Frequency Nutrition Plan
A high-frequency nutrition plan is one that leads you to your health and wellbeing goals, leaves you feeling good and does NOT include any alcohol or mind-altering substances. What are your health and wellbeing goals? You get to follow a nutrition plan or diet that is aligned with those goals. Some examples are: Mediterranean Diet, Paleo Diet, Whole 30, Vegetarian, pescatarian. You will get out of this challenge what you put into it. This means you have some latitude and flexibility when it comes to the nutrition and diet plan for the next fifty days. The only absolute no-no's are alcohol and mind-altering substances like recreational drugs and even plant medicines. Refer to High Frequency Nutrition Options at the end of this workbook and journal for more ideas.

Journaling

Follow the prompts in this workbook and journal. There is a page for each day. Start by writing the date at the top and complete the entire page in any order you see fit. Be sure to go back to the 50-Day Challenge Checklist and check off each activity once it's done.

Gratitude: Each day write down five or more things for which you are grateful. It is ok to write some of the same things down on multiple days. However, see if you can expand that list.

Intention Setting for Today: Each day write down three things that you intend on accomplishing that day. Note: The purpose is to be intentional with your attention, capacity and energy. What is required here is to write down your intentions. If you do not accomplish your intentions that day, you have still satisfied that frequency raising activity.

Give Appreciation to Someone

Each day you will acknowledge someone for making a positive difference in your life through the act of giving appreciation. Send someone an email, text, verbally share within an in-person conversation, send a letter in the mail or via a phone call. It can be a loved one, friend, neighbor, acquaintance or even a stranger. It can be something current or even from the past. You can appreciate the same person multiple times as long as you appreciate them for something different each time. You must be specific about your appreciation. It is not enough to say, "Thank you." Rather, the assignment here is to share something specific such as "I want to thank you for taking the kids to the park so I could read a book and take a bath" or "I want to let you know that I really appreciate how you always include me in the neighborhood get-togethers, it really makes me feel welcome" or in the case of a stranger "I come to this store often and you are always so upbeat, positive and smiling. It really makes me feel good when I see you and your bright smile. Thank you for being you." The key to receiving the fruit from this exercise is in being specific. Make sure to record in your journal each day, the person you acknowledged and how (text, email, phone call, written note, in person) so you can keep track and remember if you've already reached out to someone or not.

10 Minutes of Connection

Spend at least 10 minutes alone and in silence with the intention of connecting to a higher power or energy beyond yourself and your physical body. Meditation, prayer, silence with eyes closed and a genuine intention to connect will facilitate this communication and unlock inspiration that is all around you and waiting to pour into you. You can ask a question, ask for general or specific guidance or simply sit as an open receiver. Silence and eyes closed provide you with no sensatory distractions so that you can receive more clearly. Have your journal nearby to record any downloads, thoughts, inspirations, ideas or feelings you have during this connection time. Additionally, real power, growth and expansion will come from consistent, habitual, repetition of this connection and communication with a power greater than you and your physical body. Do it daily and remember, if you spend extra minutes one day, they do not roll over to the next day.

WHY TWO WORKOUTS ARE REQUIRED FOR THIS CHALLENGE

There are five main reasons why the 50-Day Challenge includes two daily workouts: one focused on strength training and the other performed outdoors. Each of these serves a unique purpose in supporting your physical, mental, emotional, and spiritual transformation.

1. Movement Prevents Stagnation

Daily movement is essential to keeping energy flowing and preventing stagnation on all levels—mental, emotional, and physical. As Napoleon Hill explained in Think and Grow Rich, success requires consistent, deliberate action. When you move your body daily, you create momentum not only in your physical state but also in your ability to take aligned action in every area of your life.

2. Strengthening Discipline and Self-Belief

Following through on a personal commitment to work out every day builds your discipline and reinforces your belief in yourself. Neville Goddard often emphasized that the foundation of manifestation is faith in your ability to align with your desired state. By honoring your workout commitment, you strengthen the bridge between thought and action, empowering your capacity to achieve anything you envision.

3. Amplifying Your Capacity for Higher Frequencies

When you engage in strength training, you strengthen not only your body but also your energetic capacity to hold higher frequencies. As you flex and tone your muscles, feel-good chemicals lying dormant within your body—such as endorphins, serotonin, dopamine, and myokines—are activated and released, raising your vibration. You can meet the 30-minute strength training requirement through exercises like push-ups, sit-ups, resistance band workouts, or lifting weights. Even everyday items, like heavy water bottles, can double as workout tools. For inspiration, YouTube offers a wealth of strength-training videos that use bodyweight or common household objects.

4. Boosting Your Mood and Well-Being

Working out releases a cocktail of "feel-good" chemicals, sometimes referred to as a "runner's high" or post-workout euphoria. These include BDNF (brain-derived neurotrophic factor), anandamide, oxytocin, and norepinephrine, which reduce stress, elevate mood, and improve cognitive function. Rhonda Byrne reminds us in The Secret that a positive emotional state is key to attracting abundance. Consistently cultivating these feel-good states through exercise has a profound cumulative effect on your overall well-being and vibration.

5. Connecting with Nature for Expansion

The outdoor workout isn't just about physical activity—it's a chance to break out of your daily norm, connect with nature, and tap into the abundance of life. Spending time outdoors expands your awareness and deepens your connection to the universal energy that sustains us all. Observing the beauty and interconnectedness of nature helps shift your mindset to one of gratitude and possibility, opening you to greater transformation.

Summary of the Two-Workout Requirement

Each day, you'll complete two 30-minute workouts. The first must be outdoors, involving movement such as running, walking, cycling, or even crawling. Set the intention to connect with nature as you move. The second workout focuses on strength training to build physical and energetic resilience.

Bonus: Yoga Counts as Strength Training

For this challenge, yoga can satisfy the 30-minute strength training requirement. Contrary to popular belief, yoga isn't merely physical exercise; it's a spiritual practice that aligns your body, mind, and spirit with universal energy. As Neville Goddard might say, yoga helps you embody the state of being that aligns with your highest potential. Plus, it fortifies your body to sustain higher levels of consciousness and frequency.

Boom—just like that, you're on your way to transformation.

THE POWER OF DAILY PERSONAL GROWTH CONTENT

As part of the 50-Day Challenge, you'll dedicate time each day to nourishing your mind and spirit with high-frequency content. You'll either read 10 pages of a non-fiction personal development or growth book or listen to 30 minutes of empowering material. This could include audiobooks, YouTube videos, podcasts, or other audio formats focused on personal development.

Why is this so essential? Think of it as "high-frequency nutrition" for your mind. Just as nutritious food fuels your body, positive and uplifting content feeds your thoughts, beliefs, and emotions. Neville Goddard taught that what we repeatedly impress upon the mind shapes our reality. By consistently immersing yourself in transformational ideas, you align your thinking with higher possibilities and expand your capacity for growth.

This practice elevates your frequency, primes your mind for success, and keeps you inspired. Whether you're learning new strategies, reframing limiting beliefs, or deepening your understanding of yourself and the world, these daily moments of intentional growth compound over time, creating profound shifts in your mindset and your life.

Every page or minute you dedicate to personal development is an investment in your transformation.

DAILY JOURNAL PROMPTS FOR REFLECTION

There is a journal prompt for a daily self-reflection assignment. Follow the prompt for that day and record your findings. Each week has a theme to the assignments, all of which are aimed at raising your frequency and building upon each other. The weekly themes are as follows:

Week 1: Awareness
Week 2: Level Up Your Language
Week 3: Identity Shifting
Week 4: Creating Space for the New
Week 5: Expansion
Week 6: Rewrite Your Stories
Week 7: Manifesting From a Higher Frequency

Use the Checklist/Program at-a-Glance to keep track of your progress and ensure that you complete each frequency raising activity each day.

Helpful tips, tricks, hacks, stacks and other ways to be efficient and optimize your experience:

Satisfying the daily 10 Minutes of Silent Alone Time

- Spend your 10 minutes of silent alone time in bed upon waking. Set your alarm for 10 minutes earlier and rather than jumping out of bed or getting on your phone or iPad, lie in bed in the hazy, sleepy state and communicate with a higher power. Ask specific questions for which you seek answers or simply ask for any information that will support your growth and expansion. Be sure to set an intention to connect to an energy and power greater than yourself.

- Spend your 10 minutes of silent alone time in bed just before going to bed. Set an alarm for 10 minutes, close your eyes and go within. I recommend doing this sitting up rather than lying completely down due to a high risk of falling asleep. Pray, meditate, or ask specific questions for which you seek answers or simply ask for any information that will support your growth and expansion. Be sure to set an intention to connect to an energy and power greater than yourself.

- If you have difficulties not having something to do during the 10 minutes of silent alone time, repeat the Ho'o Pono Pono Prayer: "I'm sorry, Please forgive me, Thank you, I love you." You can direct that prayer to someone specific, the world, Universe or cosmos. You can even direct that prayer to your body parts that are in pain or need healing.

Satisfying the daily Two 30-Minute Workouts and Consumption of Personal Development Content

- Listen to an audible book, YouTube or Podcast while walking or running outside.

- Listen to an audible book, YouTube or Podcast while strength training.

- Wear a weighted jacket, wrist or ankle weights while walking outside to satisfy the outside movement and the strength training.

Satisfying the requirement for giving appreciation:

- Have your phone and/or some note cards next to you as you fill out the gratitude section of your daily journal and workbook. When you identify gratitude for a specific person, write down that statement of gratitude then immediate text, email or write a note to that person and send it out. Now you have satisfied both requirements for that day.

- Do your workout with a partner/friend and while exercising together take a moment to look at them at the eyes and verbally share your appreciation for them in being an accountability/workout partner.

- If you do your exercise within a group fitness setting, after the class go up to the instructor and express your appreciation for them.

- While you are out in public, take a moment to look someone in the eyes and verbally express genuine gratitude for them for something specific. For example, I frequent a local Thai restaurant and one of the waiters is exceptionally friendly. I have, on several occasions, looked him in the eyes and say "Thank you for always being so upbeat and cheerful, it really makes a difference in my day."

Abstaining from alcohol and Mind-Altering Substances

- Kava tea, made from the root of the kava plant (Piper methysticum), is a popular natural remedy, especially in Pacific Island cultures. It is known for its calming and stress-relieving properties.

- Passionflower (Passiflora incarnata) is a flowering plant traditionally used for its calming and sedative properties. It is commonly consumed as a tea or tincture and offers various health benefits, primarily for stress and nervous system support

- 5-HTP (5-Hydroxytryptophan) is a naturally occurring compound that your body produces as part of serotonin synthesis. It is derived from the amino acid L-Tryptophan and is an intermediate step in the process of converting tryptophan into serotonin, a neurotransmitter that plays a significant role in mood, sleep, and appetite regulation.

- Euphoric drinks that include adaptogenic herbs, botanicals and calming agents

- Visit a local natural food store and you will find many alcohol alternatives

THE POWER OF HOʻOPONOPONO

A Practice of Forgiveness, Reconciliation, and Frequency Elevation

Hoʻoponopono (pronounced ho-oh-pono-pono) is a sacred Hawaiian practice used to restore harmony within oneself, with others, and with the world. At its heart, it's a practice of deep personal responsibility, healing, and spiritual cleansing. The word "Hoʻoponopono" roughly translates to "to make right, to correct."

This simple but profound ritual involves repeating four healing phrases:

I love you,
I'm sorry,
Please forgive me,
Thank you.

Each phrase carries a vibrational frequency that can clear emotional and energetic blockages, heal past wounds, and bring you into a state of peace, presence, and higher frequency.

Why It Works
Hoʻoponopono is based on the principle that by taking full responsibility for our inner state—our thoughts, emotions, and energy—we can transform not only ourselves but also our relationships and circumstances. When practiced consistently, it clears the mental clutter that keeps us out of alignment with joy, love, and flow.

Even if you're not consciously aware of what needs healing, the practice works on a subconscious level. It's a frequency attunement. A return to love.

How to Practice During the 50-Day Challenge

You can incorporate Hoʻoponopono into your daily practice in any of the following ways:

- **During Silent Meditation Time:** Gently repeat the four phrases silently to yourself. You may direct them toward God, yourself, someone else, a situation, or even an uncomfortable feeling. Breathe deeply, and let the energy of each phrase wash over you.

- **Before Bed or Upon Waking:** Whisper the words as a gentle daily reset. Imagine any lingering stress, resentment, or fear dissolving into light.

- **During Emotional Triggers or Resistance:** When you feel stuck, reactive, or closed off, pause and recite the phrases slowly. They help shift you out of judgment and into compassion.

- **Journaling Integration:** Write the phrases at the top of a journal page and reflect on who or what in your life might need forgiveness, gratitude, or more love. Let your hand flow without judgment.

Hoʻoponopono and Frequency

Forgiveness is one of the fastest ways to raise your frequency. When you release emotional baggage, you free up space for joy, clarity, and expansion. Let this practice be a gentle yet powerful companion to the rest of your inner work in this challenge.

Every time you say these words—**I love you, I'm sorry, Please forgive me, Thank you**—you are returning to your truth.

You are remembering who you really are.

PROGRESS ASSESSMENT FORM

This is an optional assessment form for all of the people who geek out over data (I am one of these people!) While you will most likely be experiencing all kinds of subjective outcomes, this is one way to objectively track progress.

Part 1: Frequency Baseline (Self-Assessment) Fill out BEFORE starting
Rate yourself on a scale of 1 to 10, where 1 is "very low" and 10 is "very high."

1. **Overall Life Satisfaction**: How satisfied are you with your life?

_____ / 10

2. **Energy Levels**: How much energy do you have throughout the day?

_____ / 10

3. **Emotional Well-being**: How often do you feel positive, joyful, and at peace?

_____ / 10

4. **Mental Clarity**: How clear and focused do you feel on your goals and tasks?

_____ / 10

5. **Spiritual Connection**: How connected do you feel to God/Source/Your Higher Self?

_____ / 10

6. **Alignment with Desires**: How aligned do you feel with your dreams and goals?

_____ / 10

7. **Physical Well-being**: How do you rate your physical health and fitness?

_____ / 10

8. **Self-Confidence**: How confident do you feel in your ability to create the life you desire?

_____ / 10

9. **Relationship Harmony**: How harmonious and fulfilling are your relationships?

_____ / 10

10. **Sense of Purpose**: How purposeful and meaningful does your life feel?

_____ / 10

Part 2: Habits and Practices
Answer the following:

1. Do you currently follow any daily mindfulness or gratitude practices?

☐ **Yes**   ☐ **No**

If yes, please describe briefly:

_____

2. How often do you engage in personal development (e.g., reading, workshops)?

☐ **Never**   ☐ **Occasionally**   ☐ **Regularly**

3. Describe your current physical activity routine, if any:

_____

4. What is your current diet/nutrition plan including approximate number of alcoholic drinks or other intoxicants consumed weekly?

_____

_____

5. How often do you intentionally connect with a higher power or your spiritual self?

☐ **Never**   ☐ **Occasionally**   ☐ **Regularly**

6. Do you currently track your goals or intentions daily?

☐ **Yes**   ☐ **No**

Part 3: Goals for the Program

1. What are your top 3 goals for this program?

Goal 1: _____

Goal 2: _____

Goal 3: _____

2. What are the biggest challenges or obstacles you currently face in your life?

_____

_____

_____

_____

_____

_____

3. Taking your goals from #1 a step further, describe the specific transformations you would like to see for each goal – being as specific as possible. *Example Goal 1: Lose weight – Taken a step further: Release 20 pounds of weight and be a size 6 again.*

_____

_____

_____

_____

_____

_____

POST-PROGRAM REFLECTION

(To Be Completed AFTER Day 50)

Re-rate yourself on the frequency baseline (Part 1):

1. **Overall Life Satisfaction**: How satisfied are you with your life?

    _____ / 10

2. **Energy Levels**: How much energy do you have throughout the day?

    _____ / 10

3. **Emotional Well-being**: How often do you feel positive, joyful, and at peace?

    _____ / 10

4. **Mental Clarity**: How clear and focused do you feel on your goals and tasks?

    _____ / 10

5. **Spiritual Connection**: How connected do you feel to God/Source/Your Higher Self?

    _____ / 10

6. **Alignment with Desires**: How aligned do you feel with your dreams and goals?

    _____ / 10

7. **Physical Well-being**: How do you rate your physical health and fitness?

    _____ / 10

8. **Self-Confidence**: How confident do you feel in your ability to create the life you desire?

    _____ / 10

9. **Relationship Harmony**: How harmonious and fulfilling are your relationships?

    _____ / 10

10. **Sense of Purpose**: How purposeful and meaningful does your life feel?

    _____ / 10

POST-PROGRAM REFLECTION

Which program activities had the most impact on your transformation?

_____

_____

_____

What were your biggest successes or breakthroughs?

_____

_____

_____

_____

What challenges, if any, did you face during the program, and how did you overcome them?

_____

_____

_____

_____

Do you feel more aligned with your desires and goals?

☐ **Yes**   ☐ **No**

Please explain:

_____

What will you continue to practice or implement in your life going forward?

_____

_____

_____

PREPARING FOR THE NEXT BEST VERSION OF YOU

In the space below, you're invited to step into the life you are creating. Imagine that your desires have already manifested and you are now living in the reality of your wish fulfilled.

What does an average day in this version of your life look and feel like?

Write out a full day—from the moment you wake up to when your head hits the pillow at night—in the present tense, as though it's already happening. Use "I am" statements, and express it all with gratitude, joy, and certainty.

Be as detailed as possible. Include things like:

- How do you wake up? What's the first thing you see or do?
- Where are you living? Describe your home, the surroundings, the feeling in the space.
- What kind of car (or cars) do you drive?
- Who is with you? Who do you spend time with?
- What does your physical body feel like? What are your energy levels, your vitality, your appearance?
- Where do you go for coffee, shop for food, or meet up with friends?
- What do you do for work, service, or creative expression? How do you earn income or contribute to the world?
- What brings you joy, meaning, and fulfillment throughout the day?

Let this exercise be a powerful vision-setting moment. You are not "pretending"—you are tuning in to a reality that already exists for you on a higher frequency.

Take your time, tune in with your heart, and write it all out in vivid detail.

EXAMPLE: A DAY IN THE LIFE OF MY WISH FULFILLED

I wake up naturally around 6:45 AM, feeling completely rested, energized, and grateful for another beautiful day. Sunlight filters through my linen curtains, and I stretch in my soft, spacious bed, smiling as I remember—this is my real life now.

I live in a bright, airy home by the ocean, with warm wood floors, plants in every room, and wide windows that open to the sound of waves. The air smells like salt and sunshine. I sip warm lemon water and then head out for a sunrise walk on the beach. My body feels strong, light, and vibrant. I move with ease and confidence.

Back home, I blend a smoothie filled with fresh, organic fruits and greens and sit on my balcony to journal and meditate. I affirm: I am aligned. I am thriving. I am living my purpose.

Around 9 AM, I open my laptop at my favorite little café just a few blocks from home. The staff knows me by name. I sip my iced matcha and check my messages from clients around the world. My online programs are running beautifully, and the income flows easily. I lead a 60-minute coaching call with a group of incredible women who are transforming their lives. I feel so connected, so alive.

By noon, I close my laptop and head to a nearby co-op to pick up fresh produce. I say hi to a few friends and neighbors, and then meet my partner at a rooftop bistro for lunch. We laugh, dream, and enjoy every bite.

In the afternoon, I create some new content—a podcast episode and a journal prompt for my next course. The words flow effortlessly. I work from my hammock today, and my dog snoozes beside me.

Evening is sacred. I do yoga or dance, then soak in a candlelit bath. Dinner is home-cooked, nourishing, and full of love.

Before bed, I reflect on the abundance of the day. I feel deeply fulfilled, supported by the Universe, and excited for what tomorrow brings.

I am free. I am joyful. I am abundant. I am the next best version of me.

A DAY IN THE LIFE OF
MY WISH FULFILLED

_____

_____

_____

_____

_____

_____

_____

_____

_____

_____

_____

_____

_____

_____

_____

_____

_____

_____

_____

_____

Keep Your Vision Alive

This written vision is more than just words—it's an energetic blueprint of the life you are stepping into.

Keep it close. Read it daily. Let it remind you of who you truly are and where you are headed.

At the end of your 50-day journey, consider rewriting this vision on a fresh piece of paper and carrying it with you—tucked in your journal, wallet, or pocket—as a sacred reminder.

Read it often to stay anchored in your desires, rooted in faith, and aligned with the frequency of your highest self. Let it guide you when doubt creeps in. Let it call you back when the world tries to distract you.

You are becoming. Stay connected to the truth of that.

WEEK 1

Awareness

Intentional transformation begins with awareness. Before you can shift your life, you must first become aware of your current state, patterns, and choices. This is the first step on your journey to transformation—shining a light on the areas that may need attention or realignment.

This week, you'll focus your attention and observation on becoming more mindful of yourself, your thoughts, and whether you are operating from a higher or lower frequency. Your frequency is a reflection of your energy, mindset, and patterns, and it can either align with your goals or keep you stuck in old habits.

Our frequency is influenced by seven interconnected life areas:

1. **The words we use**
2. **Our dominant thoughts**
3. **Our dominant feelings**
4. **Our beliefs**
5. **Our true desires**
6. **The actions we take (or don't take)**
7. **The choices we make**

Areas to Reflect Upon This Week:
This week, you'll place your awareness on one area each day and journal your observations without judgment. This is about pure observation, not analysis, criticism, or shame. It's an opportunity to witness yourself with compassion, curiosity, and openness. By the end of this week, you'll have built the foundation to identify patterns and intentions to help align your life with your higher self.

Remember: You are safe here. You are learning. This is not about perfection but progress. Be honest, gentle, and loving with yourself as you step into this journey.

Your Daily Journaling Exercises for This Week:
Each day this week, focus on one of the seven life areas listed above. Spend time observing and journaling about it without judgment.

Observe Your Words
How do you speak to yourself and others? Are your words affirming, supportive, and empowering? Or are they critical, limiting, or fearful?

Observe Your Dominant Thoughts
What patterns of thought seem to dominate your mental space? Are they aligned with possibility and abundance, or are they focused on fear and lack?

Observe Your Dominant Feelings
What emotions come up most often? Do you find yourself leaning into gratitude and joy, or are feelings of overwhelm, anger, or sadness more frequent?

Observe Your Beliefs
What are the core beliefs shaping your life? Do they empower you or limit you? How have they impacted your current choices?

Observe Your True Desires
Are you clear on what you truly want? Do you feel connected to your goals, or are you chasing what others expect of you?

Observe Your Actions
Are you taking consistent action toward your dreams? Which actions are supportive, and which ones are passive or fearful?

Observe Your Choices
Reflect on your daily choices. Are they coming from a place of intention, alignment, and love? Or are they reactive, habitual, or fear-based?

Each day, simply observe and record your findings. Write freely, with no judgment, shame, or expectation. These reflections are sacred moments of learning and selfdiscovery.

Key Principles to Remember This Week:

Awareness is the first step to transformation.
You can't change what you don't acknowledge. Begin by observing your patterns without judgment.

You are your own teacher and your own best friend.
Treat yourself with compassion and love through this process. You're here to grow —not to be perfect.

All transformation begins with your energy and choices.
Every thought, belief, action, and choice has a ripple effect. By observing these, you create the opportunity to consciously choose a higher frequency.

Judgment keeps you stuck; observation allows growth.
Release the need to judge yourself. Approach these observations with curiosity, kindness, and a growth mindset.

You are always growing. Every day is an opportunity to realign.
Embrace this journey knowing that growth is a process, not a destination. Every moment of awareness brings you closer to your desired life.

This week is your foundation. With each observation, you're building clarity, understanding, and the space to make intentional shifts in your life. Trust the process. You are exactly where you need to be. Let's begin.

DAY 1

Date: _____

Present Gratitude

1. _____
2. _____
3. _____
4. _____
5. _____

Intention Setting for Today

1. _____
2. _____
3. _____

Today's Reflection Assignment on Awareness

Become aware of the words you speak out loud, to yourself, type into letters, emails and write down. Refer to the back of the book for a list of High and Low Frequency Words and use the space below to record your observations of the types of words you use both high and low-frequency.

_____
_____
_____
_____

Journal space for downloads, ideas, thoughts and feelings from 10+ min connection time

_____
_____
_____
_____

Who did I send appreciation to and how (email, text, phone call, conversation, letter)?

What personal development and growth content did I consume today?

DAY 2

Date: _____

Present Gratitude

1. _____
2. _____
3. _____
4. _____
5. _____

Intention Setting for Today

1. _____
2. _____
3. _____

Today's Reflection Assignment on Awareness

Become aware of your dominant thoughts and record them here. Do these thoughts serve you? Which of your thoughts are high-frequency or low-frequency?

_____
_____
_____
_____
_____

Journal space for downloads, ideas, thoughts and feelings from 10+ min connection time

_____
_____
_____
_____

Who did I send appreciation to and how (email, text, phone call, conversation, letter)?

What personal development and growth content did I consume today?

DAY 3

Date: _____

Present Gratitude

1. _____
2. _____
3. _____
4. _____
5. _____

Intention Setting for Today

1. _____
2. _____
3. _____

Today's Reflection Assignment on Awareness

Become aware of your dominant feelings and record them here. Do these feelings serve you?
Which of your feelings are high-frequency or low-frequency?

_____
_____
_____
_____
_____

Journal space for downloads, ideas, thoughts and feelings from 10+ min connection time

_____
_____
_____
_____

Who did I send appreciation to and how (email, text, phone call, conversation, letter)?

What personal development and growth content did I consume today?

DAY 4

Date: _____

Present Gratitude

1. _____
2. _____
3. _____
4. _____
5. _____

Intention Setting for Today

1. _____
2. _____
3. _____

Today's Reflection Assignment on Awareness

Become aware of your beliefs and record them here. Do these beliefs serve you? Which of your beliefs are high-frequency or low-frequency? Example "Of course I won't get the job" vs "Of course I will get the job" or "There are no good guys in San Diego" vs "I live in ManDiego, there are guys everywhere" or "It's impossible to (fill in the blank)" vs "It's got to be possible to (fill in the blank) and I am confident I will be shown a way."

_____
_____
_____

Journal space for downloads, ideas, thoughts and feelings from 10+ min connection time

_____
_____
_____

Who did I send appreciation to and how (email, text, phone call, conversation, letter)?

What personal development and growth content did I consume today?

DAY 5

Date: _____

Present Gratitude

1. _____
2. _____
3. _____
4. _____
5. _____

Intention Setting for Today

1. _____
2. _____
3. _____

Today's Reflection Assignment on Awareness

Become aware of your true desires and record them here. This is where you really need to be honest with yourself. No judgement, just become aware of what you really want. Do YOU want this or do you think you want it because someone else really wants it for you? Use your 10 minutes of alone, connection time to ask yourself what you really desire for yourself.

_____
_____
_____

Journal space for downloads, ideas, thoughts and feelings from 10+ min connection time

_____
_____
_____
_____

Who did I send appreciation to and how (email, text, phone call, conversation, letter)?

What personal development and growth content did I consume today?

DAY 6

Date: _____

Present Gratitude

1. _____
2. _____
3. _____
4. _____
5. _____

Intention Setting for Today

1. _____
2. _____
3. _____

Today's Reflection Assignment on Awareness

Become aware of your actions and record them here. Do these actions serve you? Which of your actions are high-frequency or low-frequency?

_____
_____
_____
_____
_____

Journal space for downloads, ideas, thoughts and feelings from 10+ min connection time

_____
_____
_____
_____

Who did I send appreciation to and how (email, text, phone call, conversation, letter)?

What personal development and growth content did I consume today?

DAY 7

Date: _____

Present Gratitude

1. _____
2. _____
3. _____
4. _____
5. _____

Intention Setting for Today

1. _____
2. _____
3. _____

Today's Reflection Assignment on Awareness

Become more aware of the choices you make on a regular basis and record them here. How did your choices serve you? Which of your choices are high-frequency or low-frequency? Which choices raised your frequency? Which choices lowered your frequency?

_____
_____
_____
_____

Journal space for downloads, ideas, thoughts and feelings from 10+ min connection time

_____
_____
_____
_____

Who did I send appreciation to and how (email, text, phone call, conversation, letter)?

What personal development and growth content did I consume today?

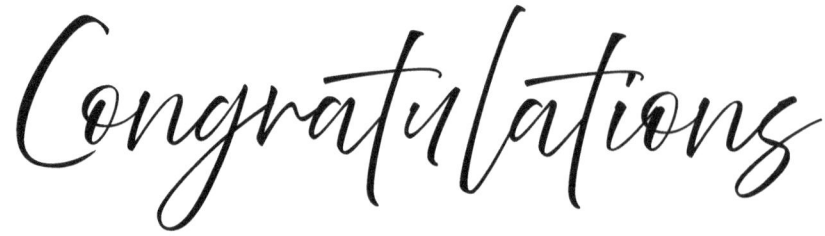

ON FINISHING WEEK 1

of this 50-Day Challenge. What did you become aware of in terms of your current state of being? Where are your areas for improvement? Record them here. In addition, what are some wins and celebrations? What changes and transformations have you observed?

You can also use this space for extra gratitude, reflections, intention setting, lists of what's going well in your life right now and so forth.

"You don't have to be great to start,
but you have to start to be great."

— Zig Ziglar

WEEK 2

Level Up Your Language

The words you use are more powerful than you may realize. They are not just sounds or random expressions—they shape your reality, your beliefs, and your experiences. Every word you speak, whether aloud or silently in your thoughts, sends signals into the quantum field, setting the manifestation process into motion. As Florence Scovel Shinn taught, *"Your words are like a boomerang, returning to you as your life experience."*

Yet, so many people remain unaware of this Universal Law. They speak from fear, doubt, or frustration without realizing that their words are shaping their reality. This week, we'll break through that unconscious pattern and start to clean up the language we use—both in our inner dialogue and external speech.

Yvonne Oswald's teachings remind us that *"every word carries energy, either raising or lowering your vibration."* This means that our words either pull us into a higher-frequency state of joy, possibility, and abundance, or keep us stuck in fear, doubt, and limitation. Our language is a direct reflection of our mindset, beliefs, and emotional state. By becoming aware of the words we use, we can consciously choose to shift toward higher-frequency language that empowers, uplifts, and aligns with our goals and dreams.

Areas to Reflect Upon This Week

This week is about more than just choosing different words—it's about developing awareness, consistency, and habit. When you intentionally shift the words you use, you can shift your vibration and, therefore, your life. This is your opportunity to observe, learn, and take control of your language to create the life you truly desire.

Your Daily Journaling Exercises for This Week

Each day this week, focus on observing and shifting your words. Journal your observations and reflections with honesty and curiosity. Here are some areas of exploration when it comes to your language:

Observe Your Spoken Words

What are the most common words you speak aloud? Are they supportive, empowering, or rooted in doubt and fear? Write them down.

Observe Your Inner Dialogue

What does your self-talk sound like? Is it kind and encouraging, or critical and limiting? Record your observations.

Notice Your Automatic Responses

Pay attention to the words that come up when you're stressed, overwhelmed, or challenged. How can you choose different words to shift your response?

Replace Fearful Words with Possibility

Take note of any fearful, doubtful, or limiting words you use. Rewrite them with possibility-focused alternatives. Example: "I can't" becomes "I can learn how."

Reframe Complaints

Observe any complaints you catch yourself making. How can you shift these into gratitude, opportunity, or affirmations? Write down or say new statements such as "Of course I will get a parking spot" or "I would love for my friend to show up on time and not gossip."

Visualize and Speak Your Desires

Write a positive affirmation or statement that reflects the life you want to create. Speak it aloud with feeling. Statements such as "Of course I will (fill in the blank)" and "I would love (fill in the blank)" are powerful and tap into the Law of Assumption taught by Neville Goddard.

Set an Intention for Your Words

Write a commitment to yourself: How will you commit to using higher-frequency language moving forward? What will you choose to focus on?

Key Principles to Remember This Week:

Your words are powerful tools of creation.
Every word you think or speak sends out instructions to the quantum field, shaping your reality.

Words are boomerangs.
What you put out into the world will return to you. Speak from a place of empowerment, gratitude, love and possibility.

Every word carries energy.
Your language either raises your vibration (joy, possibility, abundance) or lowers it (fear, doubt, lack). Choose your words wisely.

Awareness is the first step to transformation.
Notice your words without judgment. Awareness allows you to consciously choose higher-frequency alternatives rather than habitually, and often unconsciously, using low-frequency words or phrases.

Consistency builds new habits.
This week, focus on the consistent practice of shifting your language. Small, intentional changes compound into profound transformation.

Your words are your wand—use them to create magic.
Every word you speak and think is shaping your reality. Use your words to build the life you desire with love, joy, and possibility.

This week is an invitation to step into the power of your words. Shift your mindset, shift your language, and watch as your reality begins to transform. Let's begin this journey with intention, awareness, and the belief that your words have the power to create miracles.

DAY 8

Date: _____

Present Gratitude

1. _____
2. _____
3. _____
4. _____
5. _____

Intention Setting for Today

1. _____
2. _____
3. _____

Today's Reflection Assignment on Leveling Up Your Language

Look at the list of high and low-frequency words at the back of the book. Select one low-frequency word that you habitually use and replace it with a high-frequency word that you will commit yourself to using. Record your choice(s) and reflection(s) here:

_____
_____
_____
_____

Journal space for downloads, ideas, thoughts and feelings from 10+ min connection time

_____
_____
_____
_____

Who did I send appreciation to and how (email, text, phone call, conversation, letter)?

What personal development and growth content did I consume today?

DAY 9

Date: _____

Present Gratitude

1. _____
2. _____
3. _____
4. _____
5. _____

Intention Setting for Today

1. _____
2. _____
3. _____

Today's Reflection Assignment on Leveling Up Your Language

Look at the list of high and low-frequency words at the back of the book. Select another low-frequency word that you habitually use and replace it with a high-frequency word that you will commit yourself to using. Record your choice(s) and reflection(s) here:

_____
_____
_____
_____

Journal space for downloads, ideas, thoughts and feelings from 10+ min connection time

_____
_____
_____
_____

Who did I send appreciation to and how (email, text, phone call, conversation, letter)?

What personal development and growth content did I consume today?

DAY 10

Date: _____

Present Gratitude

1. _____
2. _____
3. _____
4. _____
5. _____

Intention Setting for Today

1. _____
2. _____
3. _____

Today's Reflection Assignment on Leveling Up Your Language

What are some low-frequency phrases that you habitually speak, write, think or communicate in any form? How can you switch them with higher-frequency language?.

_____
_____
_____
_____
_____

Journal space for downloads, ideas, thoughts and feelings from 10+ min connection time

_____
_____
_____
_____

Who did I send appreciation to and how (email, text, phone call, conversation, letter)?

What personal development and growth content did I consume today?

DAY 11

Date: _____

Present Gratitude

1. _____
2. _____
3. _____
4. _____
5. _____

Intention Setting for Today

1. _____
2. _____
3. _____

Today's Reflection Assignment on Leveling Up Your Language

Look at the list of high-frequency words at the back of the book. Select up to three high-frequency words and/or phrases to begin using more frequently and record them here.

_____
_____
_____
_____
_____

Journal space for downloads, ideas, thoughts and feelings from 10+ min connection time

_____
_____
_____
_____

Who did I send appreciation to and how (email, text, phone call, conversation, letter)?

What personal development and growth content did I consume today?

DAY 12

Date: _____

Present Gratitude

1. _____
2. _____
3. _____
4. _____
5. _____

Intention Setting for Today

1. _____
2. _____
3. _____

Today's Reflection Assignment on Leveling Up Your Language

Look at the list of high-frequency words at the back of the book. Select one high-frequency word to use repeatedly today. Record your choice(s) and reflection(s) here:

_____
_____
_____
_____
_____

Journal space for downloads, ideas, thoughts and feelings from 10+ min connection time

_____
_____
_____
_____

Who did I send appreciation to and how (email, text, phone call, conversation, letter)?

What personal development and growth content did I consume today?

DAY 13

Date: _____

Present Gratitude

1. _____
2. _____
3. _____
4. _____
5. _____

Intention Setting for Today

1. _____
2. _____
3. _____

Today's Reflection Assignment on Leveling Up Your Language

Observe your inner dialog today around what you tell yourself regarding your present tense, past and future. For example "I'm still broke/fat/sick/unwell/unmotivated/negative..." Replace that communication with statements like "I'm getting healthier every day" or "I'm so excited for the money and abundance that is coming my way" or "My soul mate/life partner is closer than they have ever been." Record your new inner dialog statements here and practice using them from now on.

_____
_____
_____

Journal space for downloads, ideas, thoughts and feelings from 10+ min connection time

_____
_____
_____

Who did I send appreciation to and how (email, text, phone call, conversation, letter)?

What personal development and growth content did I consume today?

DAY 14

Present Gratitude

1. _____
2. _____
3. _____
4. _____
5. _____

Intention Setting for Today

1. _____
2. _____
3. _____

Today's Reflection Assignment on Leveling Up Your Language

Where or when do you find yourself naturally using high-frequency language and where or when do you find yourself using low-frequency words and phrases? Is this an internal dialog, external dialog or both?

_____
_____
_____
_____

Journal space for downloads, ideas, thoughts and feelings from 10+ min connection time

_____
_____
_____
_____

Who did I send appreciation to and how (email, text, phone call, conversation, letter)?

What personal development and growth content did I consume today?

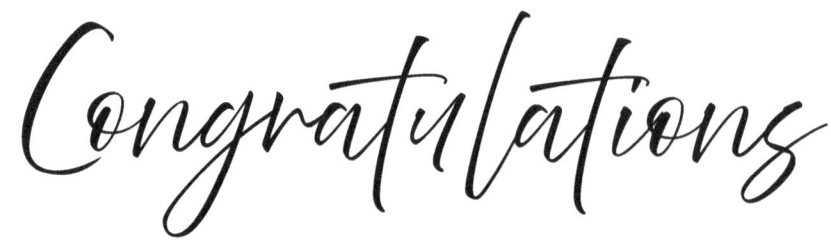

Congratulations

ON FINISHING WEEK 2

of this 50-Day Challenge. What are some wins and celebrations?
What changes and transformations have you observed?

You can also use this space for extra gratitude, reflections, intention setting,
lists of what's going well in your life right now and so forth.

"Raise your words, not your voice. It is
rain that grows flowers, not thunder."

— Rumi

WEEK 3
Identity Shifting

It has been said, *"We don't get what we want. We get what we are."* This means that who you are—your identity—attracts more of the same into your life. If you desire a soulmate, financial freedom, an ideal body, or any other goal, you must first embody the identity of the person who already has those things.

At first, this can feel like a paradox—like the chicken and the egg: *What comes first, being or having?* The answer lies in **shifting your identity.** Identity shifting is the process of becoming a match for your desires by transforming your mindset, habits, beliefs, and actions to align with the person you're striving to become.

When you step into this higher version of yourself, you're sending a clear signal to the Universe. You're telling it that you're ready to receive your desires, but it begins with embodying the essence of who you want to become *right now*

This week, you'll learn how to shift your identity by taking ownership of your current state and aligning it with the person you truly desire to become. Remember: **Every small action counts.** Identity shifting isn't about perfection—it's about taking consistent baby steps toward embodying the traits, habits, and beliefs of your highest self.

Areas to Reflect Upon This Week:

1. Become Aware & Honest About Your Current Identity:
Begin by observing your thoughts, feelings, habits, and routines. Ask yourself: *Who am I right now? Are there aspects of myself that no longer align with the life I want to create?* Awareness is the first step toward transformation. Once you acknowledge aspects that can grow or shift, you can begin the journey toward change.

2. Identify the Traits & Habits of the Identity You Desire:
Visualize the person you want to become: *What does their mindset look like? What are their daily habits? How do they speak, act, and interact with the world?* Write these down. This is the blueprint of your desired self.

3. Take Daily Action to Embody That Identity Now:
Ask yourself: *What can I do today to embody that person?* Examples: If you want to be a best-selling author, commit to writing for 30 minutes every day. Act as if you already are that person. Actions build momentum, even if they start small.

Your Daily Journaling Exercises for This Week:
Over the next seven days, you'll journal each day to reflect on your journey of identity shifting. Use these prompts to bring awareness and intentional action to your transformation:

Who do you want to be in the world?
Write about the person you are striving to become. How would this version of you show up in all areas of life?

What one thing can you do today to step into that identity?
Choose one small action that aligns with your desired self and commit to doing it today

What habits, thoughts, or beliefs are keeping you stuck?
Reflect on what you may need to let go of to shift your identity and step into your power.

What traits or qualities would someone embodying your ideal identity possess?
Write a list of these traits. How can you cultivate them in your daily life?

How would the person you want to become handle fear, challenges, or setbacks?
Visualize your desired self responding to challenges with strength, confidence, and faith.

What's one way you can invest in yourself to embody this new identity?
Think about learning, personal development, choices, or habits that can signal commitment to your transformation.

What would you do today if you knew you were already the person you want to become?
Write this as if you're already stepping into this new identity.

How would your relationships, environment, and daily routines change if you fully embodied this new identity?
Reflect on what aspects of your life would shift and how you could create alignment with your higher self.

Who would you surround yourself with if you were living as your highest self?
Consider the people, groups, or environments you might choose to connect with and explore how to start seeking these connections.

What are you grateful for as you step into this transformation?
Gratitude is an essential part of manifestation and transformation. Write about the positive aspects of this journey and how far you've come.

Key Principles to Remember This Week:

You attract what you are, not just what you want.
Embodying the identity you desire sends the energetic signal to the Universe to align your experiences with that frequency.

Awareness is the first step to change.
Notice your current thoughts, patterns, and habits without judgment. Acknowledging them is empowering.

Small actions lead to big transformations.
Every small step you take toward becoming the person you desire strengthens your new identity.

You can choose to act as if right now.
Your actions can shift your mindset and habits, creating the person you want to become today.

Your identity is flexible and malleable.
Just because you've been a certain way in the past doesn't mean you can't shift, evolve, and become someone new.

DAY 15

Date: _____

Present Gratitude

1. _____
2. _____
3. _____
4. _____
5. _____

Intention Setting for Today

1. _____
2. _____
3. _____

Today's Reflection Assignment on Identity Shifting

Who do you want to be in the world? What one thing will you do today to be that person now?

_____
_____
_____
_____
_____

Journal space for downloads, ideas, thoughts and feelings from 10+ min connection time

_____
_____
_____
_____

Who did I send appreciation to and how (email, text, phone call, conversation, letter)?

What personal development and growth content did I consume today?

DAY 16

Date: _____

Present Gratitude

1. _____
2. _____
3. _____
4. _____
5. _____

Intention Setting for Today

1. _____
2. _____
3. _____

Today's Reflection Assignment on Identity Shifting

If you were living your dream life, having achieved your top 3 goals identified at the beginning of this program, how would you go about your day?

_____
_____
_____
_____
_____

Journal space for downloads, ideas, thoughts and feelings from 10+ min connection time

_____
_____
_____

Who did I send appreciation to and how (email, text, phone call, conversation, letter)?

What personal development and growth content did I consume today?

DAY 17

Date: _____

Present Gratitude

1. _____
2. _____
3. _____
4. _____
5. _____

Intention Setting for Today

1. _____
2. _____
3. _____

Today's Reflection Assignment on Identity Shifting

If you were living your dream life, having achieved your top 3 goals identified at the beginning of this program, how would spend your money?

_____
_____
_____
_____
_____
_____

Journal space for downloads, ideas, thoughts and feelings from 10+ min connection time

_____
_____
_____
_____

Who did I send appreciation to and how (email, text, phone call, conversation, letter)?

What personal development and growth content did I consume today?

DAY 18

Date: _____

Present Gratitude

1. _____
2. _____
3. _____
4. _____
5. _____

Intention Setting for Today

1. _____
2. _____
3. _____

Today's Reflection Assignment on Identity Shifting

If you were living your dream life, having achieved your top 3 goals identified at the beginning of this program, how would you dress on a regular basis?

_____
_____
_____
_____
_____

Journal space for downloads, ideas, thoughts and feelings from 10+ min connection time

_____
_____
_____
_____

Who did I send appreciation to and how (email, text, phone call, conversation, letter)?

What personal development and growth content did I consume today?

DAY 19

Date: _____

Present Gratitude

1. _____
2. _____
3. _____
4. _____
5. _____

Intention Setting for Today

1. _____
2. _____
3. _____

Today's Reflection Assignment on Identity Shifting

If you were living your dream life, having achieved your top 3 goals identified at the beginning of this program, with whom would you spend your work time and free time?

_____
_____
_____
_____
_____
_____

Journal space for downloads, ideas, thoughts and feelings from 10+ min connection time

_____
_____
_____
_____

Who did I send appreciation to and how (email, text, phone call, conversation, letter)?

What personal development and growth content did I consume today?

DAY 20

Date: _____

Present Gratitude

1. _____
2. _____
3. _____
4. _____
5. _____

Intention Setting for Today

1. _____
2. _____
3. _____

Today's Reflection Assignment on Identity Shifting

If success was guaranteed, and you could be anything you wanted to be – how would you contribute to society/work/create/invest/live your life?

_____
_____
_____
_____
_____

Journal space for downloads, ideas, thoughts and feelings from 10+ min connection time

_____
_____
_____
_____

Who did I send appreciation to and how (email, text, phone call, conversation, letter)?

What personal development and growth content did I consume today?

DAY 21

Date: _____

Present Gratitude

1. _____
2. _____
3. _____
4. _____
5. _____

Intention Setting for Today

1. _____
2. _____
3. _____

Today's Reflection Assignment on Identity Shifting

If you were given 10 million dollars tax free today, how would that change your identity? Your goals? Your work/career/contribution to society?

_____
_____
_____
_____
_____

Journal space for downloads, ideas, thoughts and feelings from 10+ min connection time

_____
_____
_____
_____

Who did I send appreciation to and how (email, text, phone call, conversation, letter)?

What personal development and growth content did I consume today?

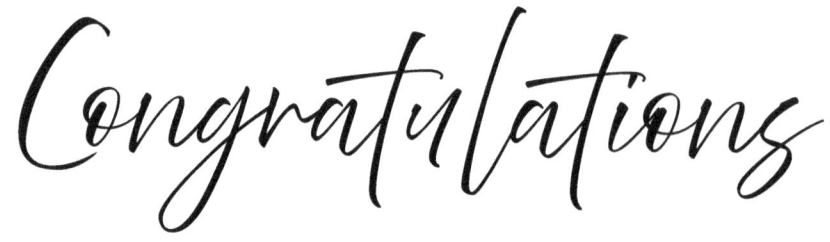

Congratulations

ON FINISHING WEEK 3

of this 50-Day Challenge. What are some wins and celebrations?
What changes and transformations have you observed?

You can also use this space for extra gratitude, reflections, intention setting,
lists of what's going well in your life right now and so forth.

"Your life is a reflection of your identity.
Shift your thoughts, change your beliefs,
and you shift your entire reality."

— Neville Goddard

WEEK 4
Creating Space for the New

As your frequency and energy rise, you may begin to notice that certain people, places, situations, or material possessions no longer align with the elevated, authentic version of you. Neville Goddard taught that *"to create a new reality, we must first embody the consciousness of the life we desire."* Holding on to remnants of the *"old you"* can anchor you to past patterns and limitations, making it more challenging to step fully into the future you're creating.

This week, you'll focus on the powerful and transformative act of **purging**—letting go of what no longer serves your highest good. This isn't just about physical decluttering (though that's part of it); it's about creating energetic space to invite new opportunities, blessings, and possibilities into your life. As Florence Scovel Shinn reminds us, *"Nature abhors a vacuum."* When you clear away the old—whether material, emotional, or energetic—the Universe has the opportunity to rush in and fill that space with new opportunities aligned with your higher frequency.

This week is also a journey of releasing old attachments, outdated habits, draining relationships, and mental clutter. As you do this, you make way for transformation, growth, and alignment with the life you desire. Let's step into this process with gratitude, trust, and faith.

Areas to Reflect on This Week:
Here are key areas to focus on as you declutter your life and create space for the new:

Material Possessions: Go through your belongings and release anything that feels heavy, outdated, or no longer serves a purpose. Ask yourself: *Does this item spark joy?* (Inspired by Marie Kondo's philosophy.) If it doesn't align with your current vibration, let it go with gratitude.

People and Relationships: Evaluate your connections. Are there relationships that feel draining, toxic, or no longer support your growth? Purging isn't about cutting ties recklessly but about consciously choosing to maintain relationships that *uplift* and *support* your evolution.

Habits, Places, and Situations: Look at your routines, your environment, and the commitments you've made. Ask yourself: *Do these reflect the person I'm becoming?* If not, consider how you can release, shift, or transform them to better align with your goals.

Inner Purge: Release outdated beliefs, fears, doubts, and attachments that no longer serve you. Neville Goddard emphasized, *"Imagination creates reality."* Letting go of mental clutter makes room for new, empowering thoughts and beliefs to take root.

Your Daily Journaling Exercises for This Week:
Each day this week, dedicate time to both physical and emotional decluttering.
Reflect on your observations and intentions as you clear space in your life. You will
be releasing the old and thereby inviting in the new for these areas of your life:

Physical Declutter
Take time to go through a physical space in your home. Which items no longer
resonate with you or your current vision?
Let them go with gratitude, knowing they are making room for new opportunities.

Evaluate Relationships
Write about the people in your life. Which relationships feel supportive? Which feel
draining?
Set an intention to nurture relationships that align with your growth and perform a
"friends cleanse" where needed.

Walk Away From Routines and Environments
Reflect on the routines and environments you've created. Do they match your goals
and dreams? If not, create a plan to shift them.

Releasing Old Beliefs
Write down beliefs or thoughts that have held you back. Reframe them into
affirmations of growth and possibility.

Key Principles to Remember This Week:

Purging is an act of faith.
Letting go of the old signals to the Universe that you trust in the abundance of new possibilities.

You create space for what you desire.
Whether through decluttering your physical space or releasing outdated emotions and beliefs, clearing makes room for transformation and growth.

Energetic space is just as important as physical space.
By addressing fears, doubts, and limiting beliefs, you make room for higher-frequency thoughts and opportunities.

Change begins with letting go.
Trust in the process. Every item, relationship, or belief you release creates new space for blessings and growth.

Gratitude amplifies your shifts.
As you let go, express gratitude for each release. This shifts your vibration and aligns you with abundance.

This week, allow yourself the freedom of releasing what no longer serves you. Trust the process of clearing out physical, emotional, and mental clutter. With each item, belief, or habit you release, you're signaling to the Universe that you're ready for growth, transformation, and new possibilities. You are stepping into a higher-frequency life— lighten your load and trust in the journey.

DAY 22

Date: _____

Present Gratitude

1. _____
2. _____
3. _____
4. _____
5. _____

Intention Setting for Today

1. _____
2. _____
3. _____

Today's Reflection Assignment on Creating Space for the New

Go through your closets and drawers and remove items that you no longer use, leave you with bad feelings or do not bring you joy. You will repeat this step for three days this week. What did you release today?

_____
_____
_____
_____

Journal space for downloads, ideas, thoughts and feelings from 10+ min connection time

_____
_____
_____
_____

Who did I send appreciation to and how (email, text, phone call, conversation, letter)?

What personal development and growth content did I consume today?

DAY 23

Date: _____

Present Gratitude

1. _____
2. _____
3. _____
4. _____
5. _____

Intention Setting for Today

1. _____
2. _____
3. _____

Today's Reflection Assignment on Creating Space for the New

Go through your closets and drawers and remove items that you no longer use, leave you with bad feelings or do not bring you joy. You will repeat this step for three days this week. What did you release today?

_____
_____
_____
_____

Journal space for downloads, ideas, thoughts and feelings from 10+ min connection time

_____
_____
_____
_____

Who did I send appreciation to and how (email, text, phone call, conversation, letter)?

What personal development and growth content did I consume today?

DAY 24

Date: _____

Present Gratitude

1. _____
2. _____
3. _____
4. _____
5. _____

Intention Setting for Today

1. _____
2. _____
3. _____

Today's Reflection Assignment on Creating Space for the New

Go through your closets and drawers and remove items that you no longer use, leave you with bad feelings or do not bring you joy. Collect all of the items from the past three days, express gratitude for these items and then release these items today by either donating, trashing or giving them away. What items did you release in this process of making space for the new?

_____
_____
_____

Journal space for downloads, ideas, thoughts and feelings from 10+ min connection time

_____
_____
_____
_____

Who did I send appreciation to and how (email, text, phone call, conversation, letter)?

What personal development and growth content did I consume today?

DAY 25

Date: _____

Present Gratitude

1. _____
2. _____
3. _____
4. _____
5. _____

Intention Setting for Today

1. _____
2. _____
3. _____

Today's Reflection Assignment on Creating Space for the New

Write out a lists of relationships in your life. Next to the name of that relationship place a + or –. Commit yourself to either improving the "-" relationships or limiting your exposure to them or eliminating them completely. Our relationships add to our frequency. If you can clear out negative relationships, you can create space for new, positive ones to enter your life.

_____
_____
_____

Journal space for downloads, ideas, thoughts and feelings from 10+ min connection time

_____
_____
_____
_____

Who did I send appreciation to and how (email, text, phone call, conversation, letter)?

What personal development and growth content did I consume today?

DAY 26

Date: _____

Present Gratitude

1. _____
2. _____
3. _____
4. _____
5. _____

Intention Setting for Today

1. _____
2. _____
3. _____

Today's Reflection Assignment on Creating Space for the New

This is another chance to write out a list of relationships in your life. Next to the name of that relationship place a + or −. Commit yourself to either improving the "-" relationships or limiting your exposure to them or eliminating them completely. Our relationships add to our frequency. If you can clear out negative relationships, you can create space for new, positive ones to enter your life.

_____
_____
_____

Journal space for downloads, ideas, thoughts and feelings from 10+ min connection time

_____
_____
_____
_____

Who did I send appreciation to and how (email, text, phone call, conversation, letter)?

What personal development and growth content did I consume today?

DAY 27

Date: _____

Present Gratitude

1. _____
2. _____
3. _____
4. _____
5. _____

Intention Setting for Today

1. _____
2. _____
3. _____

Today's Reflection Assignment on Creating Space for the New

Write out a list of environments in your life where you spend a good amount of time. Next to the name of that environment place a + or –. Commit yourself to limiting your exposure to or eliminating completely the environments with "-". Our environments add to our frequency. If you can clear out negative environments, you can create space for new, positive ones to enter your life.

_____
_____
_____

Journal space for downloads, ideas, thoughts and feelings from 10+ min connection time

_____
_____
_____
_____

Who did I send appreciation to and how (email, text, phone call, conversation, letter)?

What personal development and growth content did I consume today?

DAY 28

Date: _____

Present Gratitude

1. _____
2. _____
3. _____
4. _____
5. _____

Intention Setting for Today

1. _____
2. _____
3. _____

Today's Reflection Assignment on Creating Space for the New

Here is another opportunity to transform your environments. List them out and place a + or – next to that environment. Commit yourself to limiting your exposure to or eliminating completely the environments with "-". Our environments add to our frequency. If you can clear out negative environments, you can create space for new, positive ones to enter your life.

_____
_____
_____

Journal space for downloads, ideas, thoughts and feelings from 10+ min connection time

_____
_____
_____
_____

Who did I send appreciation to and how (email, text, phone call, conversation, letter)?

What personal development and growth content did I consume today?

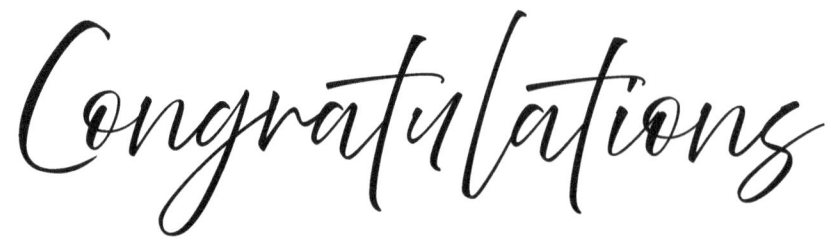

Congratulations

ON FINISHING WEEK 4

of this 50-Day Challenge. What are some wins and celebrations?
What changes and transformations have you observed?

You can also use this space for extra gratitude, reflections, intention setting,
lists of what's going well in your life right now and so forth.

"Nature abhors a vacuum, and when you empty your life of clutter—be it physical, emotional, or spiritual—you create space for the good you desire to flow in."

— Florence Scovel Shinn

WEEK 5
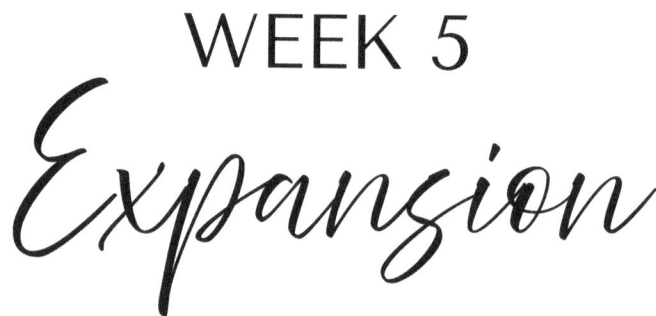
Expansion

Mantra for this week and beyond: **"There is nothing wrong. There is nothing to fix."**

This week is an invitation to step into the spacious energy of **growth, possibility, and transformation**. Expansion doesn't come from fixing what's "wrong"—it comes from recognizing that everything is unfolding perfectly to support your evolution.

When we judge or resist our current reality, we anchor ourselves to limitation. But when we release the need to fix and instead choose to expand, we open to infinite potential. Let this week be about softening into what is while holding a bold, loving vision for what could be.

In alignment with the teachings of **Neville Goddard, Napoleon Hill**, and **Rhonda Byrne**, you are reminded that the universe is **abundant, limitless, and responsive**. What you focus on grows. When you direct your energy toward expansion—rather than correction—you activate the creative power of the divine within you.

Psychologist **Carol Dweck's** work on growth mindset further supports this idea: true transformation comes when we welcome challenge, release judgment, and appreciate every experience as part of our soul's unfolding.

Expansion is not about striving. It's about allowing.
It's not about force. It's about flow.
It's not about fixing. It's about **remembering** who you really are.

Areas to Reflect Upon This Week:

This week, explore any area of your life that feels stuck, heavy, or resistant. Instead of judging or trying to fix it, approach it with **loving awareness** and ask:

What might this be asking me to expand into?
What's the higher version of this experience?
How can I shift from contraction to possibility?

Your Daily Journaling Exercises for This Week:
Each day this week, take time to reflect and write in your journal using these types of prompts:

Where are you "fixing," and where can you focus on growing instead?
Identify areas where you've been trying to fix problems or control outcomes. How can you shift your energy toward growth, learning, and expansion in these areas?

Choose an area of your life you don't like. Ask yourself: What would I love to happen here?
Write about the ideal outcome with vivid detail, imagining it as if it has already come to pass.

Where are you judging, and how can you move into gratitude?
Reflect on where you've been judgmental—toward yourself, others, or circumstances. How can you reframe this judgment into gratitude? What can you appreciate about the situation, even if it's challenging?

Key Principles to Remember This Week:

Energy flows where attention goes.
Focus on expansion, not limitation.

Gratitude is the gateway to abundance.
Judgment contracts, but gratitude expands.

Imagination is creation.
See yourself already living the life you desire and feel the emotions that accompany it.

This week is your opportunity to stretch your mindset and elevate your energy. Embrace the power of your imagination and gratitude as tools to expand your reality. Remember, as Napoleon Hill said, *"Whatever the mind can conceive and believe, it can achieve."* Let's grow together!

DAY 29

Present Gratitude

1. _____
2. _____
3. _____
4. _____
5. _____

Intention Setting for Today

1. _____
2. _____
3. _____

Today's Reflection Assignment on Expansion

Where are you "fixing" and where can you focus on growing instead?

_____
_____
_____
_____
_____
_____

Journal space for downloads, ideas, thoughts and feelings from 10+ min connection time

_____
_____
_____
_____

Who did I send appreciation to and how (email, text, phone call, conversation, letter)?

What personal development and growth content did I consume today?

DAY 30

Date: _____

Present Gratitude

1. _____
2. _____
3. _____
4. _____
5. _____

Intention Setting for Today

1. _____
2. _____
3. _____

Today's Reflection Assignment on Expansion

Write out a positive statement around receiving more money into your life. Example "I am open to receiving more financial abundance/wealth/money/prosperity into my life. You may want to write this out several times and feel into this statement.

_____
_____
_____
_____

Journal space for downloads, ideas, thoughts and feelings from 10+ min connection time

_____
_____
_____
_____

Who did I send appreciation to and how (email, text, phone call, conversation, letter)?

What personal development and growth content did I consume today?

DAY 31

Date: _____

Present Gratitude

1. _____
2. _____
3. _____
4. _____
5. _____

Intention Setting for Today

1. _____
2. _____
3. _____

Today's Reflection Assignment on Expansion

Write out a positive statement around receiving more love into your life. Example "I am open to receiving and experiencing more love in all of the relationships of my life." You may want to write an additional statement that is more relationship specific as well such as "I am open to receiving and experiencing a deeper sense of love and gratitude with my [fill in the blank.]

_____
_____
_____
_____

Journal space for downloads, ideas, thoughts and feelings from 10+ min connection time

_____
_____
_____
_____

Who did I send appreciation to and how (email, text, phone call, conversation, letter)?

What personal development and growth content did I consume today?

DAY 32

Date: _____

Present Gratitude

1. _____
2. _____
3. _____
4. _____
5. _____

Intention Setting for Today

1. _____
2. _____
3. _____

Today's Reflection Assignment on Expansion

Where are you "fixing" and where can you focus on growing instead?

_____
_____
_____
_____
_____

Journal space for downloads, ideas, thoughts and feelings from 10+ min connection time

_____
_____
_____
_____

Who did I send appreciation to and how (email, text, phone call, conversation, letter)?

What personal development and growth content did I consume today?

DAY 33

Date: _____

Present Gratitude

1. _____
2. _____
3. _____
4. _____
5. _____

Intention Setting for Today

1. _____
2. _____
3. _____

Today's Reflection Assignment on Expansion

Where are you judging? How can you move into gratitude and away from this judgement?

_____
_____
_____
_____
_____

Journal space for downloads, ideas, thoughts and feelings from 10+ min connection time

_____
_____
_____
_____

Who did I send appreciation to and how (email, text, phone call, conversation, letter)?

What personal development and growth content did I consume today?

DAY 34

Date: _____

Present Gratitude

1. _____
2. _____
3. _____
4. _____
5. _____

Intention Setting for Today

1. _____
2. _____
3. _____

Today's Reflection Assignment on Expansion

Identify an area of your life that you do not like. What would you love to happen here?

_____
_____
_____
_____
_____

Journal space for downloads, ideas, thoughts and feelings from 10+ min connection time

_____
_____
_____
_____

Who did I send appreciation to and how (email, text, phone call, conversation, letter)?

What personal development and growth content did I consume today?

DAY 35

Date: _____

Present Gratitude

1. _____
2. _____
3. _____
4. _____
5. _____

Intention Setting for Today

1. _____
2. _____
3. _____

Today's Reflection Assignment on Expansion

Re-examine that area of your life that you do not like from yesterday. What would you love to happen here? Record your ideal outcome here again.

_____
_____
_____
_____
_____

Journal space for downloads, ideas, thoughts and feelings from 10+ min connection time

_____
_____
_____
_____

Who did I send appreciation to and how (email, text, phone call, conversation, letter)?

What personal development and growth content did I consume today?

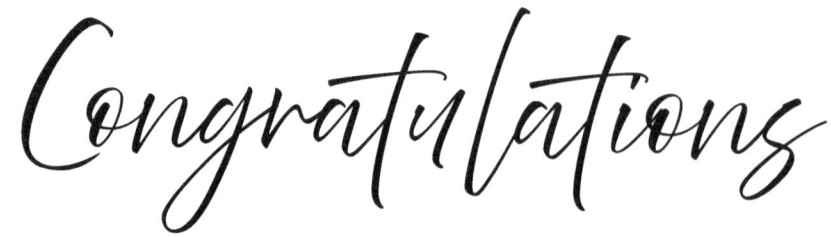

Congratulations

ON FINISHING WEEK 5

of this 50-Day Challenge. What are some wins and celebrations?
What changes and transformations have you observed?

You can also use this space for extra gratitude, reflections, intention setting,
lists of what's going well in your life right now and so forth.

"Feeling is the secret. Assume the feeling of your wish fulfilled, and it must be realized."

— Neville Goddard

WEEK 6
Rewrite Your Stories

Your story has the power to shape your reality. The narrative you tell yourself about your life creates the lens through which you experience the world. As Neville Goddard taught, *"Imagination creates reality,"* and the stories we choose to focus on determine the reality we manifest. If you find yourself stuck in a cycle of repeating a not-so-positive story, this week is your opportunity to rewrite it—to transform your perspective, to release judgment, and to step into a more empowering and expansive version of your life.

Drawing from *The Master Key System, The Secret, and Think and Grow Rich*, we know that by shifting our mindset and focusing on growth rather than limitation, we shift our frequency and align ourselves with abundance and transformation. This week, you'll engage with the concept of *Gifts for Growth*—the idea that even our hardest moments, setbacks, and challenges are opportunities in disguise. They're not just obstacles; they are the stepping stones to personal growth, strength, and transformation.

Carol Dweck's *Mindset* emphasizes the power of adopting a growth-oriented perspective, recognizing that every challenge can lead to learning and empowerment if we choose to see it that way. This week, you'll practice rewriting your stories to reflect this growth mindset—transforming limiting beliefs into opportunities for appreciation, healing, and self-discovery.

Areas to Reflect on This Week

1. Where in your life are you holding onto a story that feels limiting or disempowering?
2. How can you see this story as part of your journey rather than a stumbling block?
3. What moments from your past could you reframe to find the hidden Gifts for Growth?
4. What would your life look like if you fully embraced the belief that everything happening is for your ultimate growth and expansion?

As you reflect on these areas, remember that transformation begins with awareness. By exploring these questions and embracing a new narrative, you are paving the way for a more aligned, empowered, and abundant version of yourself.

Your Daily Journaling Exercises for This Week:
Each day this week, you'll complete the following prompts as a part of your journey to rewrite your stories:

Identify a Story:
Reflect on a story from your life that feels not-so-positive. This could be a past experience, relationship, decision, or pattern that you've found yourself revisiting or struggling with.

Rewrite in a New Light:
With no judgment, rewrite this story in a more empowering, positive way. See it as part of your journey, without shame or guilt. Focus on the growth and lessons learned, not the pain or suffering.

Recognize the Gifts for Growth:
Every setback, hardship, or challenge carries the potential for transformation. Acknowledge and express gratitude for these moments by identifying the Gifts for Growth they brought into your life. What did you learn? How did they shape you?

Reframe with Appreciation:
Use statements of appreciation to shift your perspective. Examples could be:
"I am grateful for this experience because it taught me resilience."
"This challenge was a catalyst for me to discover my inner strength."
"I appreciate the lessons this moment offered and how it has led me to growth."
"Rejection is often God's protection."

Key Principles to Remember This Week:

Your story has the power to shape your present and future.
Choose to rewrite it with empowerment, hope, and possibility.

Setbacks are not failures; they are opportunities.
Gifts for Growth transform pain into lessons, hardship into strength, and struggle into understanding.

Judgment creates resistance; compassion creates freedom.
Rewrite your stories without judgment and with appreciation for the wisdom you've gained.

This week, commit to freeing yourself from the old stories that no longer serve you. As you shift your narrative, you shift your vibration and open the door to a new, empowered version of your life.

As Rhonda Byrne shares in *The Power*, *"The more you focus on the positive, the more positivity will flow into your life."* You have the power to transform your story. Let's begin.

DAY 36

Date: _____

Present Gratitude

1. _____
2. _____
3. _____
4. _____
5. _____

Intention Setting for Today

1. _____
2. _____
3. _____

Today's Reflection Assignment on Rewriting Your Life Stories

Identify a story from your life that is not-so-positive and you find yourself repeating often. Rewrite this story here in a more positive light, with no judgement and use statements of appreciation for the Gifts for Growth you received:

_____
_____
_____
_____

Journal space for downloads, ideas, thoughts and feelings from 10+ min connection time

_____
_____
_____

Who did I send appreciation to and how (email, text, phone call, conversation, letter)?

What personal development and growth content did I consume today?

DAY 37

Date: _____

Present Gratitude

1. _____
2. _____
3. _____
4. _____
5. _____

Intention Setting for Today

1. _____
2. _____
3. _____

Today's Reflection Assignment on Rewriting Your Life Stories

Identify a story from your life that is not-so-positive and you find yourself repeating often. You can repeat the story from yesterday or select another one. Rewrite this story here in a more positive light, with no judgement and use statements of appreciation for the Gifts for Growth you received:

_____
_____
_____
_____

Journal space for downloads, ideas, thoughts and feelings from 10+ min connection time

_____
_____
_____
_____

Who did I send appreciation to and how (email, text, phone call, conversation, letter)?

What personal development and growth content did I consume today?

DAY 38

Date: _____

Present Gratitude

1. _____
2. _____
3. _____
4. _____
5. _____

Intention Setting for Today

1. _____
2. _____
3. _____

Today's Reflection Assignment on Rewriting Your Life Stories

Identify a story from your life that is not-so-positive and you find yourself repeating often. You can repeat the story from yesterday or select another one. Rewrite this story here in a more positive light, with no judgement and use statements of appreciation for the Gifts for Growth you received:

_____
_____
_____
_____

Journal space for downloads, ideas, thoughts and feelings from 10+ min connection time

_____
_____
_____
_____

Who did I send appreciation to and how (email, text, phone call, conversation, letter)?

What personal development and growth content did I consume today?

DAY 39

Date: _____

Present Gratitude

1. _____
2. _____
3. _____
4. _____
5. _____

Intention Setting for Today

1. _____
2. _____
3. _____

Today's Reflection Assignment on Rewriting Your Life Stories

Identify a story from your life that is not-so-positive and you find yourself repeating often. You can repeat the story from yesterday or select another one. Rewrite this story here in a more positive light, with no judgement and use statements of appreciation for the Gifts for Growth you received:

_____
_____
_____
_____

Journal space for downloads, ideas, thoughts and feelings from 10+ min connection time

_____
_____
_____
_____

Who did I send appreciation to and how (email, text, phone call, conversation, letter)?

What personal development and growth content did I consume today?

DAY 40

Date: _____

Present Gratitude

1. _____
2. _____
3. _____
4. _____
5. _____

Intention Setting for Today

1. _____
2. _____
3. _____

Today's Reflection Assignment on Rewriting Your Life Stories

Notice a story you tell about yourself that begins with phrases like "I've always been…", "That's just how I am," or "This is how my life goes." Gently question this story: Is it absolutely true? Rewrite this story from the perspective of the highest version of yourself. Describe who you are now choosing to be, how you respond differently, and how this new story supports the life you are building.

_____
_____
_____
_____

Journal space for downloads, ideas, thoughts and feelings from 10+ min connection time

_____
_____
_____
_____

Who did I send appreciation to and how (email, text, phone call, conversation, letter)?

What personal development and growth content did I consume today?

DAY 41

Present Gratitude

1. _____
2. _____
3. _____
4. _____
5. _____

Intention Setting for Today

1. _____
2. _____
3. _____

Today's Reflection Assignment on Rewriting Your Life Stories

Bring to mind a story you have been carrying that once protected you or helped you make sense of something difficult. This may be a story about why something didn't work out, why you had to be strong, or why you learned to hold back. Now ask yourself: "Do I still need this story to feel safe or understood?" Rewrite the story as a closing chapter— honoring what it gave you, and consciously choosing a new story that reflects who you are becoming and how you want to move forward.

_____
_____
_____

Journal space for downloads, ideas, thoughts and feelings from 10+ min connection time

_____
_____
_____

Who did I send appreciation to and how (email, text, phone call, conversation, letter)?

What personal development and growth content did I consume today?

DAY 42

Date: _____

Present Gratitude

1. _____
2. _____
3. _____
4. _____
5. _____

Intention Setting for Today

1. _____
2. _____
3. _____

Today's Reflection Assignment on Rewriting Your Life Stories

Think about a story you have rewritten or are in the process of rewriting this week. Now look for evidence —past or present—that supports this new story. For example: Moments where you acted differently, choices you made that reflect growth, situations where you showed strength, courage, or clarity. Write about at least three pieces of evidence that prove this new story is already taking root in your life.

_____
_____
_____

Journal space for downloads, ideas, thoughts and feelings from 10+ min connection time

_____
_____
_____
_____

Who did I send appreciation to and how (email, text, phone call, conversation, letter)?

What personal development and growth content did I consume today?

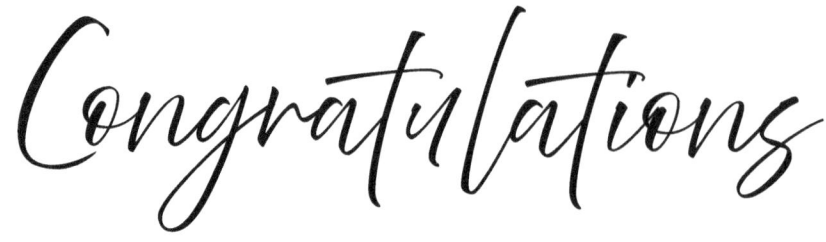

ON FINISHING WEEK 6

of this 50-Day Challenge. What are some wins and celebrations?
What changes and transformations have you observed?

You can also use this space for extra gratitude, reflections, intention setting,
lists of what's going well in your life right now and so forth.

"Change your thoughts and
you change your world."

— Norman Vincent Peale

WEEK 7

Manifesting From a Higher Frequency

A **high-frequency** is a magnet for all forms of abundance—money, love, joy, and opportunities from the Universe. The truth is: *Anything you desire can be yours*. If you have a desire, it means that you have also been given the ability to manifest it. Your desires are not random; they are divinely placed within you, and the Universe has already set the stage for their fulfillment.

This week, we'll focus on **maintaining high-frequency activities** while beginning to *plant the seeds* of manifestation with unwavering faith, trust, and belief. Manifestation is simpler than most people think. As the ancient truth states: *"Ask and ye shall receive."* However, the key to manifestation lies in the belief that you will receive it. Believing isn't just hoping —it's having faith that your desire is already yours and aligning your thoughts, feelings, and actions with that belief. This requires conscious focus, trust in the process, and the willingness to remove the internal and external obstacles standing in your way.

This week, you'll focus on **one central desire** to manifest. It can be as small or as big as you like—*it's your desire, and you are meant to have it*. Each day, you will write about this desire, your thoughts on faith, belief, trust, and the obstacles you may encounter as you align with your manifestation.

You'll continue this process for **eight days straight**, with the understanding that manifestation is a journey that requires consistency and perseverance. Many give up just before the magic happens. Bigger desires take time, patience, and faith—but know this: the **God/the Universe/Source/Creator/Divine Intelligence is eager to bless you with your desires.** Your job is simply to clear the obstacles that are blocking the flow.

Are you ready to step into the most exciting part of this journey? You have the power to create a life beyond your wildest dreams. Trust the process, believe, and let's get started!

Areas to Reflect on This Week

1. What is one desire that excites you, but also feels slightly out of reach?

2. Where in your life do you notice doubt or fear holding you back from fully believing in your ability to manifest this desire?

3. How would your thoughts and actions shift if you knew with certainty that your manifestation is already on its way?

4. What daily practices or habits can you commit to this week to keep your frequency high and your faith strong?

Reflection creates clarity, and clarity is the foundation of manifestation. By exploring these questions, you'll strengthen your alignment with your desire and open yourself to receive the abundance waiting for you.

Your Daily Journaling Exercises for This Week:

Over the next eight days, you'll engage in daily journaling to focus on one main thing you want to manifest. Here's how:

Define Your Desire

Write down one main thing you want to manifest. It can be anything— money, love, a new career, better health, or inner peace. Write it down with clarity and detail.

Reflect on Your Faith

Ask yourself: Do I truly believe this is possible? Write about your current feelings toward this desire and examine where faith may be lacking.

Trust the Process

Journal about trust. Are you willing to let go of control and trust the Universe to bring your desire to you? Write about any fears or doubts that may be standing in the way.

Identify the Obstacles

Write about any thoughts, fears, or circumstances that you perceive as obstacles. Acknowledge them without judgment and commit to releasing them.

Shift Your Mindset

Using affirmations, write out new statements that shift your mindset toward abundance. Examples: "I trust that God/the Universe/Divine Intelligence is working to bring me my desire or something even better" or "I am worthy of all the blessings coming to me."

Visualize Your Desire

Take time to visualize your life as though your desire has already manifested. Journal about the feelings, thoughts, and experiences you'll have when it becomes reality.

Observe the Signs

Write about any synchronicities, feelings, or signs you notice as you move through this process. Are the doors opening? Trust in these moments.

Reaffirm Your Desire

Write your desire again. Reaffirm your faith and trust in the process. Know that every word and thought you put toward your manifestation is powerful.

Key Principles to Remember This Week:

Your desires are divinely placed within you.
Trust that if you have a desire, you also have the ability to manifest it.

Faith is the currency of manifestation.
Believing that your desires are already yours shifts your vibration and aligns you with the flow of abundance.

Obstacles are opportunities for growth.
Examine your fears, doubts, or limitations with compassion and release them to create space for your manifestations.

Consistency is essential.
Journaling every day for eight days (or beyond) creates momentum and maintains focus on your desire.

The Universe is eager to give to you.
Trust that you are supported by the Divine, and every step you take toward your desire is bringing you closer to it.

Let go and trust the process.
Surrendering the "how" allows the Universe to bring your desire to you in the best possible way.

Remember: *You are a magnet for abundance when you align with a higher frequency and trust the process of manifestation.* Your words, thoughts, and emotions are creating your reality—stay focused, persistent, and open to the blessings that await. Are you ready to manifest your dreams? Let's go!

"Create the vision, trust the process, and embody the energy of your dreams— because the universe aligns with the unstoppable force of a soul on fire."

DAY 43

Date: _____

Present Gratitude

1. _____
2. _____
3. _____
4. _____
5. _____

Intention Setting for Today

1. _____
2. _____
3. _____

Today's Reflection Assignment on Manifesting from a Higher Frequency

What is one thing you really want to manifest? Write it down as though you already have it. A great example is this: "I am so happy and grateful now that I have (enter your desire in the present tense). As you write it, observe and record any thoughts or feelings that arise. What thoughts and feelings support and serve this desire? Which thoughts and feelings do not and need to be released, replaced and removed? Do this every day for the remainder of this challenge and until that desire manifests.

_____
_____
_____

Journal space for downloads, ideas, thoughts and feelings from 10+ min connection time

_____
_____
_____
_____

Who did I send appreciation to and how (email, text, phone call, conversation, letter)?

What personal development and growth content did I consume today?

DAY 44

Date: _____

Present Gratitude

1. _____
2. _____
3. _____
4. _____
5. _____

Intention Setting for Today

1. _____
2. _____
3. _____

Today's Reflection Assignment on Manifesting from a Higher Frequency

Write down the one thing you want to manifest in present tense, as though you already have it. Write down how having this thing makes you feel. Does having this thing make you feel safe, loved, seen, accomplished, fulfilled?

_____
_____
_____
_____

Journal space for downloads, ideas, thoughts and feelings from 10+ min connection time

_____
_____
_____
_____

Who did I send appreciation to and how (email, text, phone call, conversation, letter)?

What personal development and growth content did I consume today?

DAY 45

Date: _____

Present Gratitude

1. _____
2. _____
3. _____
4. _____
5. _____

Intention Setting for Today

1. _____
2. _____
3. _____

Today's Reflection Assignment on Manifesting from a Higher Frequency

Write down the one thing you want to manifest as you have been, in the present tense, as though you have it. Example: "I am so happy and grateful now that I have [enter the thing]. And having [enter the thing] makes me feel so [enter the feelings].

_____
_____
_____
_____

Journal space for downloads, ideas, thoughts and feelings from 10+ min connection time

_____
_____
_____
_____

Who did I send appreciation to and how (email, text, phone call, conversation, letter)?

What personal development and growth content did I consume today?

DAY 46

Date: _____

Present Gratitude

1. _____
2. _____
3. _____
4. _____
5. _____

Intention Setting for Today

1. _____
2. _____
3. _____

Today's Reflection Assignment on Manifesting from a Higher Frequency

Write down the one thing you are manifesting once again. Include present tense, as though it is already yours, how grateful you to have become the type of person who has this thing and how having it makes you feel.

_____
_____
_____
_____

Journal space for downloads, ideas, thoughts and feelings from 10+ min connection time

_____
_____
_____
_____

Who did I send appreciation to and how (email, text, phone call, conversation, letter)?

What personal development and growth content did I consume today?

DAY 47

Date: _____

Present Gratitude

1. _____
2. _____
3. _____
4. _____
5. _____

Intention Setting for Today

1. _____
2. _____
3. _____

Today's Reflection Assignment on Manifesting from a Higher Frequency

Continue to write down the one thing you are manifesting as though you have it already, how it makes you feel and express gratitude for being given it (even if it hasn't arrived yet).

_____
_____
_____
_____
_____

Journal space for downloads, ideas, thoughts and feelings from 10+ min connection time

_____
_____
_____
_____

Who did I send appreciation to and how (email, text, phone call, conversation, letter)?

What personal development and growth content did I consume today?

DAY 48

Date: _____

Present Gratitude

1. _____
2. _____
3. _____
4. _____
5. _____

Intention Setting for Today

1. _____
2. _____
3. _____

Today's Reflection Assignment on Manifesting from a Higher Frequency

Write a description of who you are now that you have this dream or desire. Image who you need to be to have the one thing you are manifesting. Get into as much detail as possible and include how becoming this person makes you feel.

_____
_____
_____
_____

Journal space for downloads, ideas, thoughts and feelings from 10+ min connection time

_____
_____
_____
_____

Who did I send appreciation to and how (email, text, phone call, conversation, letter)?

What personal development and growth content did I consume today?

DAY 49

Date: _____

Present Gratitude

1. _____
2. _____
3. _____
4. _____
5. _____

Intention Setting for Today

1. _____
2. _____
3. _____

Today's Reflection Assignment on Manifesting from a Higher Frequency

Write a thank you letter to God/the Universe/Divine Intelligence, expressing gratitude for receiving your desire/wish – even if it hasn't shown up. Example "Thank you so much for giving me [enter your dream and desire] by [date or time frame]. This gift allows me to feel [enter your feelings] and I am forever grateful for this gift and open to receiving these gifts and more."

_____
_____
_____

Journal space for downloads, ideas, thoughts and feelings from 10+ min connection time

_____
_____
_____

Who did I send appreciation to and how (email, text, phone call, conversation, letter)?

What personal development and growth content did I consume today?

DAY 50

Date: _____

Present Gratitude

1. _____
2. _____
3. _____
4. _____
5. _____

Intention Setting for Today

1. _____
2. _____
3. _____

Today's Reflection Assignment on Manifesting from a Higher Frequency

Write out the one thing you are manifesting, the person you will have become to achieve this dream/desire and how it makes you feel. Continue this practice beyond the 50 days and make sure to fill out the page of reflection on a day in the life of the wish fulfilled included in this workbook.

_____
_____
_____
_____

Journal space for downloads, ideas, thoughts and feelings from 10+ min connection time

_____
_____
_____
_____

Who did I send appreciation to and how (email, text, phone call, conversation, letter)?

What personal development and growth content did I consume today?

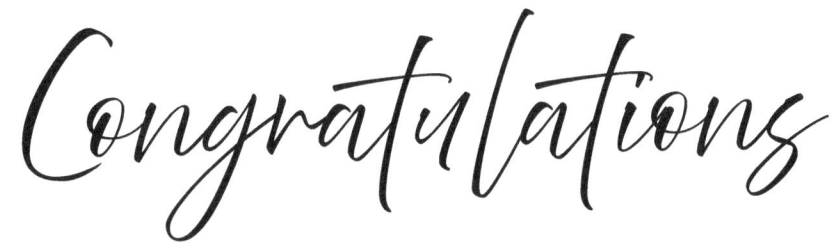

ON FINISHING WEEK 7

of this 50-Day Challenge. What are some wins and celebrations? What changes and transformations have you observed? Use the next few blank pages to continue your reflection.

You can also use this space for extra gratitude, reflections, intention setting, lists of what's going well in your life right now and so forth.

"When you align your thoughts and actions with a higher frequency, you become a magnet for miracles, abundance, and all that you desire."

— Napoleon Hill

HEALTHY NUTRITION PLANS

Here are some popular diet and nutrition plans that are designed to improve overall health and well-being and align well with health-focused programs like this one:

1. Whole30
A 30-day elimination diet designed to reset your eating habits and identify food sensitivities.
- Focus: Whole, unprocessed foods.
- Allowed: Vegetables, fruits, lean proteins, nuts, seeds, and healthy fats.
- Avoid: Added sugars, alcohol, grains, legumes, dairy, and processed foods.
- Purpose: Reduces inflammation, improves digestion, and promotes better energy and focus.

2. Mediterranean Diet
Inspired by the traditional eating habits of countries bordering the Mediterranean Sea.
- Focus: Balance and variety of nutrient-rich foods.
- Includes: Vegetables, fruits, whole grains, lean proteins (fish and poultry), olive oil, nuts, seeds, and limited dairy.
- Limits: Red meat, processed foods, and refined sugars.
- Purpose: Supports heart health, reduces chronic disease risk, and promotes longevity.

3. Paleo Diet
Modeled after the dietary patterns of ancient hunter-gatherers.
- Focus: Natural, unprocessed foods.
- Includes: Meat, fish, vegetables, fruits, nuts, and seeds.
- Excludes: Grains, dairy, legumes, processed foods, and added sugars.
- Purpose: Reduces inflammation and supports weight management.

4. Low-Carb/High-Fat (Keto)
A high-fat, moderate-protein, and very low-carb diet aimed at achieving ketosis.
- Focus: Shifting the body's energy source from glucose to fat.
- Includes: Fatty fish, meat, eggs, cheese, nuts, seeds, non-starchy vegetables, and healthy oils.
- Avoids: Sugary foods, grains, starchy vegetables, and most fruits.
- Purpose: Promotes fat loss, improves insulin sensitivity, and increases mental clarity.

5. Clean Eating
A flexible approach focused on eating minimally processed foods.
- Focus: Balanced, nutrient-dense meals.
- Includes: Fresh produce, lean proteins, whole grains, healthy fats, and natural sweeteners like honey.
- Avoids: Refined sugars, artificial ingredients, and heavily processed foods.
- Purpose: Enhances energy, digestion, and overall health.

6. Intermittent Fasting (IF)

A timing-based eating approach rather than a specific food list.

- Focus: Cycling between eating and fasting periods.
- Popular Methods:
  16:8 (16-hour fast, 8-hour eating window).
  5:2 (5 days of regular eating, 2 days of reduced calorie intake).
- Purpose: Supports weight management, improves metabolic health, and reduces inflammation.

7. Plant-Based Diet

Primarily focuses on foods derived from plants, with optional inclusion of animal products in moderation.

- Focus: Nutrient-dense, plant-derived foods.
- Includes: Vegetables, fruits, legumes, nuts, seeds, and whole grains.
- Excludes (optional): Meat, dairy, and processed foods.
- Purpose: Improves heart health, reduces environmental impact, and supports overall wellness.

8. Anti-Inflammatory Diet

Designed to reduce chronic inflammation in the body.

- Focus: Foods that combat inflammation.
- Includes: Leafy greens, berries, fatty fish, olive oil, turmeric, and ginger.
- Avoids: Refined carbs, sugary drinks, fried foods, and processed meats.
- Purpose: Supports joint health, reduces chronic pain, and promotes overall vitality.

9. DASH Diet (Dietary Approaches to Stop Hypertension)

A heart-healthy eating plan designed to prevent and lower high blood pressure.

- Focus: Reducing sodium and increasing nutrient-rich foods.
- Includes: Fruits, vegetables, whole grains, lean proteins, and low-fat dairy.
- Limits: High-sodium foods, sweets, and red meat.
- Purpose: Improves cardiovascular health and supports weight loss.

10. Macros-Based Nutrition (Flexible Dieting)

Focuses on tracking macronutrient intake (protein, fats, and carbs) rather than specific foods.

- Focus: Meeting daily macronutrient targets.
- Includes: Any foods that fit your macronutrient goals.
- Purpose: Offers flexibility while supporting fitness and body composition goals.

These plans can complement a health-focused program, but it's essential to choose one that aligns with your goals, preferences, and lifestyle for long-term success. If needed, consult a nutritionist to tailor a plan that works best for you!

HIGH-FREQUENCY WORDS

These words and phrases promote love, joy, gratitude, empowerment and connection:

Gratitude & Abundance

- Grateful
- Thankful
- Appreciation
- Overflow
- Receiving
- Generosity
- Blessed
- Prosperity
- Fulfilled
- Openness
- Abundant
- Overflowing
- Divine provision
- Receiving with ease
- I am grateful now
- More than enough
- Infinite supply
- Magnet for miracles
- I am richly blessed
- I welcome abundance

Love & Connection

- Love
- Unconditional love
- Connected
- Heart-centered
- Compassion
- Affection
- Loving presence
- Acceptance
- Belonging
- Soul family
- Divine union
- Sacred bonds
- Kindness
- Forgiveness
- I am loved
- I love freely
- Open-hearted
- Deep connection
- I choose love
- Love is who I am

Peace & Serenity

- Peace
- Tranquility
- Ease
- Calm
- Flow
- Stillness
- Surrender
- Presence
- Letting go
- Trust
- Harmonious
- Gentle
- Balanced
- Inner quiet
- I am at peace
- In the now
- Free from worry
- Safe and secure
- Centered
- Divine timing

HIGH-FREQUENCY WORDS

Joy & Enthusiasm

- Joy
- Bliss
- Radiant
- Enthusiastic
- Exuberant
- Playful
- Delight
- Uplifted
- Inspired
- Alive
- Vibrant
- Laughing
- Cheerful
- Ecstatic
- Celebrating
- I am joy
- Every moment is a gift
- Sparkling with energy
- Fun and free
- Lighthearted

Spiritual & Inspirational

- Divine
- Source
- Sacred
- Infinite
- Eternal
- Connected
- Higher self
- Aligned
- Inspired
- Guided
- Wisdom
- Inner knowing
- Light
- Truth
- Oneness
- Awakened
- Transcendent
- Expansion
- Ascension
- I am divine

Positive Action

- Inspired action
- Momentum
- Aligned effort
- Progress
- Movement
- Flowing forward
- Clarity
- Purposeful
- Directed
- Persistent
- Engaged
- Committed
- Courageous
- Decisive
- Empowered action
- I move forward
- I take aligned steps
- Everything supports me
- I show up fully
- I choose growth

HIGH-FREQUENCY WORDS

Empowerment & Strength

- Strong
- Capable
- Empowered
- Resilient
- Confident
- Bold
- Unstoppable
- Tenacious
- Fearless
- Victorious
- Inner power
- Steadfast
- Rising
- Warrior of light
- I am powerful
- I claim my strength
- I create my reality
- I rise higher
- Rooted and rising
- Brave

Motivation & Momentum

- Driven
- Motivated
- Determined
- Inspired
- Focused
- Ambitious
- Disciplined
- Unwavering
- Passionate
- Hungry for more
- I stay the course
- I embrace challenges
- Every day I grow
- I am unstoppable
- Forward focused
- Determined to thrive
- I ignite my potential
- I fuel my dreams
- Momentum is mine
- I keep going

Alignment & Receiving

- Aligned
- Receiving
- Allowing
- Effortless
- Magnetic
- Synchronicity
- In flow
- Worthy
- Deserving
- Open
- I receive with grace
- Life supports me
- It's already done
- I surrender and trust
- Available
- Receptive
- Supported
- Unfolding
- Mission-Driven
- Heart-Centered

LOW-FREQUENCY WORDS

Low frequency words can evoke fear, anger, guilt and/or other low emotional states.
Here is a list of low-frequency words and phrases with high-frequency alternatives.

Fear & Anxiety Transmuted

Low Frequency ➡️ **Higher Frequency Reframe**

Low Frequency	Higher Frequency Reframe
afraid	"I choose to feel safe in this moment."
anxious	"I trust that everything is working out for me."
worry	"I replace worry with faith."
nervous	"I am prepared and supported."
scared	"I move forward with courage."
dread	"I open to new possibilities with hope."
panic	"I breathe and come back to my center."
insecure	"I remember my inner power."
hesitant	"I act with clarity and confidence."
uneasy	"I choose peace in uncertainty."
restless	"I am calm and present."
suspicious	"I trust that life is for me."
trapped	"I am free to choose differently."
threatened	"I am protected by divine grace."
vulnerable	"My openness is my strength."
avoid	"I face what's in front of me with strength."
paralyzed	"I take one small step forward."
apprehensive	"I welcome what's next with readiness."

LOW-FREQUENCY WORDS

Low frequency words can evoke fear, anger, guilt and/or other low emotional states. Here is a list of low-frequency words and phrases with high-frequency alternatives.

Anger & Hostility Transmuted

Low Frequency ➤ **Higher Frequency Reframe**

- angry
- resentful
- bitter
- annoyed
- irritated
- judgmental
- furious
- hate
- I hate this/that/him/her

- "I allow myself to release and return to peace."
- "I choose forgiveness for my own freedom."
- "I let go so I can grow."
- "I choose patience and perspective."
- "I allow grace to guide my response."
- "I honor each soul's journey, including mine."
- "I transmute fire into focused action."
- "I release what hardens my heart."
- "This isn't a good fit for me right now"

Guilt & Shame Transmuted

Low Frequency ➤ **Higher Frequency Reframe**

- guilty
- ashamed
- regretful
- embarrassed
- unworthy
- remorseful
- disgraced

- "I make amends and move forward with love."
- "I accept myself fully and grow from this."
- "I'm grateful for what I've learned."
- "I embrace my humanness with compassion."
- "I am enough, just as I am."
- "I choose healing over punishment."
- "I realign with my truth and begin again."

LOW-FREQUENCY WORDS

Low frequency words can evoke fear, anger, guilt and/or other low emotional states. Here is a list of low-frequency words and phrases with high-frequency alternatives.

Sadness & Despair Transmuted

Low Frequency ➤ **Higher Frequency Reframe**

Low Frequency	Higher Frequency Reframe
• sad	• "I honor this emotion and let it move through me."
• depressed	• "I welcome the light back into my life."
• hopeless	• "Even now, hope is possible."
• broken	• "I am healing and becoming whole."
• grief	• "I allow love to hold my sorrow."
• empty	• "I invite in fullness and purpose."
• abandoned	• "I am deeply connected and loved."
• problem	• "I see an opportunity for growth here."

Lack & Limitation Transmuted

Low Frequency ➤ **Higher Frequency Reframe**

Low Frequency	Higher Frequency Reframe
• poor	• "I am rich in creativity and possibility."
• broke	• "I am resourceful and open to abundance."
• stuck	• "I am evolving, one step at a time."
• stupid	• "I am/they are learning and growing."
• blocked	• "I'm realigning to let things flow."
• not enough	• "I am more than enough."
• deprived	• "I receive all that I need in divine timing."
• struggling	• "I'm learning how to thrive."

INFLUENCES AND ADDITIONAL RESOURCES:

This workbook is inspired by the wisdom of many incredible thinkers and authors in the manifestation, personal development and growth space, including:

Yvonne Oswald, PhD *(Every Word Has Power)*

Florence Scovel Shinn *(The Game of Life and How to Play It and The Magic Path of Intuition)*

Marie Kondo *(The Life-Changing Magic of Tidying Up: The Japanese Art of Decluttering and Organizing)*

Neil Donald Walsh *(Happier Than God)*

Napolean Hill *(Think and Grow Rich)*

Carol S. Dweck *(Mindset)*

Gabby Bernstein *(The Universe Has Your Back, May Cause Miracles, Super Attractor and more!)*

Rhonda Byrne *(The Secret, The Magic, The Power and The Greatest Secret)*

Neville Goddard *(The Complete Reader)*

Bob Proctor and his teachings on the Law of Attraction and Manifestation

Charles F. Haanel *(The Master Key System)*

Joe Vitale *(Zero Limits: The Secret Hawaiian System for Wealth, Health, Peace and More)*

Louise Hay *(You Can Heal Your Life)*

Esther and Jerry Hicks *(Ask and It Is Given)*

Pamela Serure *(The 3-Day Energy Fast)*

Gay Hendricks (The Big Leap)

Michael Singer (Untethered Soul and Surrender Experiment)

Norman Vincent Peale (The Power of Positive Thinking)

REFLECTION SPACE

for Your Experiences While Completing this 50-Day Challenge

REFLECTION SPACE

for Your Experiences While Completing this 50-Day Challenge

REFLECTION SPACE

for Your Experiences While Completing this 50-Day Challenge

REFLECTION SPACE

for Your Experiences While Completing this 50-Day Challenge

REFLECTION SPACE

for Your Experiences While Completing this 50-Day Challenge

REFLECTION SPACE

for Your Experiences While Completing this 50-Day Challenge

_____

_____

_____

_____

_____

_____

_____

_____

_____

_____

_____

_____

_____

_____

_____

_____

_____

_____

_____

_____

_____

_____

_____

_____

_____

REFLECTION SPACE

for Your Experiences While Completing this 50-Day Challenge

STAYING TETHERED TO THE NEXT BEST VERSION OF YOU

In the space below, you're invited to once again step into the next-level life you are creating.

Imagine that your dreams and desires have already manifested and you are now living in the reality of your wish fulfilled.

What does an average day in this version of your life look and feel like?

Write out a full day—from the moment you wake up to when your head hits the pillow at night—in the present tense, as though it's already happening. Use "I am" statements, and express it all with gratitude, joy, and certainty.

Be as detailed as possible.

Include things like: How do you wake up? What's the first thing you see or do? Where are you living? Describe your home, the surroundings, the feeling in the space. What kind of car do you drive? Who is with you? Who do you spend time with? What does your physical body feel like? What are your energy levels, your vitality, your appearance? Where do you go for coffee, shop for food, or meet up with friends? What do you do for work, service, or creative expression? How do you earn income or contribute to the world? What brings you joy, meaning, and fulfillment throughout the day? Let this exercise be a powerful vision-setting moment. You are not "pretending"—you are tuning in to a reality that already exists for you on a higher frequency. Take your time, tune in with your heart, and write it all out in vivid detail.

A DAY IN THE LIFE OF
MY WISH FULFILLED

Keep shining your light!